Critical Thinking in Nursing

Case Studies Across the Curriculum

Carol J. Green, PhD, RN, ARNP

Johnson County Community College

Overland Park, Kansas

Instructor's Annotated Edition

PRENTICE HALL HEALTH

Upper Saddle River, New Jersey 07458

Senior Project Editor:	Virginia Simione Jutson
Associate Editor:	Stephanie Kellogg
Managing Editor:	Wendy Earl
Publishing Assistants:	Susan Teahan, Peggy Hammett
Production Editor:	David Novak
Text and Cover Design:	Brad Greene, Greene Design
Printer/Binder:	Courier
Cover Photography:	James Gritz

© 2000 by Prentice-Hall, Inc.
Upper Saddle River, New Jersey 07458

10 9 8 7 6 5

ISBN 0-8053-8538-X

Prentice-Hall International (UK) Limited, London
Prentice-Hall of Australia Pty. Limited, Sydney
Prentice-Hall Canada Inc., Toronto
Prentice-Hall Hispanoamerica, S.A., Mexico
Prentice-Hall of India Private Limited, New Delhi
Prentice-Hall of Japan, Inc., Tokyo

CONTRIBUTORS

Joanna M. Basuray, RN, PhD
Towson University
Towson, Maryland

Pamela Baxter, RN, BA, BScN
McMaster University
Hamilton, Ontario
Canada

Barbara Byrd, RN, MSN
Hocking Technical College
Nelsonville, Ohio

Anita Finkelman, RN, MSN
Resources for Excellence
University of Cincinnati
Cincinnati, Ohio

Sammie Justeson, RN, BSN, CCRN
Internet Communications Corporation
    of America
Logan, Utah

Penny L. Marshall, RN, PhD
Johnson County Community College
Overland Park, Kansas

REVIEWERS

Karen Burke, RN, MS
Clatsop Community College
Astoria, Oregon

Jane Freeman, RN, MSN, EdD
Jacksonville State University
Jacksonville, Alabama

Diana Hankes, RN, PhD
Columbia College
Milwaukee, Wisconsin

Kim Welch Hoover, RN, MSN
Alcorn State University
Natchez, Mississippi

Linda North, RN, MSN, EdS
Athens Area Technical Institute
Athens, Georgia

Sue Orshan, RNC, PhD, FACCE
Woman's Health Consultant
Princeton, New Jersey

Golden Tradewell, RN, MSN
McNeese State University
Lake Charles, Louisiana

Judith Wilkinson, RNC, PhD, ARNP
Johnson County Community College
Overland Park, Kansas

About the Author

Dr. Carol J. Green is a frequent speaker to nursing faculty and practitioners on the subject of critical thinking. She is currently on the nursing faculty of Johnson County Community College in Kansas, where she teaches critical care and perioperative clinical nursing, renal, immunology, and critical care didactic nursing. She is the author of several publications and computer programs, including the *Student Study Guide and Instructor's Manual for Phipp's Medical Surgical Nursing* (Mosby) and *Case Studies on Multiple Sclerosis* (Health Sciences Consortium). Dr. Green is a Commander in the United States Navy Nurse Corps, Reserve.

Acknowledgments

I wish to thank my contributors for the time and effort they put forth in writing many of the cases used in this workbook: Dr. Joanna Basuray, Pam Baxter, Barbara Byrd, Dr. Penny Marshall-Chura, Anita Finkelman, and Sammie Justesen. I am also grateful to my reviewers for theirs comments and suggestions, especially Dr. Judith Wilkinson.

Special appreciation and thanks are due to Stephanie Kellogg, Associate Editor, and Ginnie Simione Jutson, Senior Project Editor, for their patience, suggestions, and keeping me on track.

A very special thanks to my family: daughters Kathy and Debi, grandchildren Jessica, Mathew, and Luke, dogs Katie, Mollie, and Mandy, cats Sammy and Missy, and most importantly, my husband Chuck Nigro for giving up evenings, weekends, walks, movies, dinners, and so on, so that I could complete this project and reach one of my personal goals. I love you all.

Preface

This workbook will help you practice critical thinking through the analysis of nursing case studies. As with the typical nursing curriculum, the cases encompass several nursing specialties in a variety of hospital, clinical, and community settings. Each of the client case studies present a unique diagnosis and situation for the nursing student to analyze. Along with the variety presented, each case requires a combination of attitude and cognitive critical thinking components. A few of the cases, however, emphasize one type of thinking over the other because of the subject matter.

You may be asked by your instructor to complete one or more of these case studies as part of your classroom work, clinical work, or as a make-up assignment. Sometimes you will complete a case study independently, and other times you might work in a group with other students. Regardless of how you use the workbook, the following guidelines will help you obtain maximum benefit from it.

Completing the Practice Sessions

Read the introduction to the workbook and complete the *Critical Thinking Practice Ses-*sions that follow. These activities will acquaint you with the concepts and language of critical thinking and will help you separate attitudes from cognitive critical thinking skills. These activities will also prepare you to complete the exercises for each of the case studies.

Case Studies

The case studies in this workbook pertain to a variety of the specialty areas of nursing, including adult health nursing, community and home care nursing, maternal-newborn nursing, pediatric nursing, and mental health nursing. Many of the case studies overlap, and your instructor may assign a case study from one section even though your class is studying a different specialty. For example, one of the *Mental Health Nursing* case studies involves a nurse completing a home care admission assessment on a client who has been diagnosed with paranoid schizophrenia. Although it is in the *Mental Health Nursing* section, the setting of this case study is in the community, thus it can be studied as a community and home care nursing case. Along with the occasional combining of the nurse specialties listed above, gerontology is incorporated into a few of the *Community and Home Care, Adult Health Nursing,* and *Mental Health Nursing* case studies as well.

Critical Thinking Questions

You can use the strategies outlined in the Introduction to answer all of the critical thinking questions in this workbook. There is sufficient data included in each case study to direct your learning. You may, however, need to research specific nursing care, pathophysiology, drug effects, and so on, in order to fully answer some of the questions. This workbook is not based on a specific textbook, therefore you can choose (or your instructor can assign) any textbook or reference book to help answer the case study questions. With some questions, the prioritized framework provided by your school or institution can be used as a source. The nature of critical thinking questions is that there are no definitive and exact answers; however, suggested activities to help address the questions are provided in the *Instructor's Annotated Edition* of this workbook.

The last question of each case study asks, "What attitude and cognitive critical thinking components did you use to address this case?" This question is particularly beneficial in that it encourages you to think about and identify your own critical thinking processes. To answer this question, you must consider each of the critical thinking components presented in the Introduction, and then determine how you used those components to answer the questions posed in the case study. For example, in answering the question, "What are the priority nursing diagnoses for this client?" use the cognitive components of clustering data and identifying patterns and compare the client's data with the defining characteristics of the nursing diagnosis you have selected.

Nursing Process

The nursing process has been integrated throughout the workbook, and it is an excellent vehicle—when used appropriately—to promote critical thinking. The case studies in this workbook can also be used in conjunction with a nursing process text, such as *Nursing Process: A Critical Thinking Approach* by Judith Wilkinson, to help you learn how to use the nursing process effectively.

Critical Thinking and Nursing Education

I believe that critical thinking should be included in all aspects of nursing education. These case studies are based on critical thinking theory, use critical thinking language, and foster critical thinking when used as suggested. I hope that the workbook will provide you with case studies that allow you to learn and practice critical thinking in your nursing career. You will be surprised at how quickly you will learn critical thinking language and use higher order thinking.

Sample Case Study with Suggested Activities

Urinary Tract Infection

The client is an 84-year-old retired auto worker with a history of two myocardial infarctions and coronary artery bypass surgery 2 years ago. He has had numerous problems since his cardiac surgery. He does not eat well and his *fluid intake is less than 1000 mls per day*. He has a history of *urinary retention* and requires the use of an *indwelling urinary catheter*. His wife cares for him at home, and he receives visits from the home health care nurse every 4 weeks.

During a routine morning visit, the nurse notices that there is only *150 mL of urine in the urinary drainage bag*. His wife states that she *hasn't emptied the bag since last evening around 6:00 PM*. The client's *urine is cloudy, dark gold in color, and has a strong odor*. The nurse also observes a small amount of *purulent drainage from the client's urethra*. He complains of *mild low back pain*, which he attributes to lying in bed too long. His blood pressure is 130/90, heart rate 98 and regular, respiratory rate 20 and regular, and temperature *100.8F* orally. The nurse changes the client's urinary catheter and obtains a urine specimen. After calling the physician, she draws blood for a CBC and differential.

1. What conclusions can you draw about the client's situation based on the data provided?

   a. Separate normal from abnormal data. In this case study, the abnormal data is *printed in italics*.

   b. Cluster data into related categories, analyzing for pattern(s).

   "…indwelling urinary catheter…"

   "…150 mL urine output since 6:00 PM…"(it is now morning)   Data shows

   "…urine is cloudy, dark, …[with] strong odor…"   altered urinary

   "…purulent drainage from urethra…"   pattern consistent

   "…complains of…low back pain…"   with infection

   "…temperature 100.8F orally…"

c. Compare manifestations commonly associated with a urinary tract infection (UTI) with the client's data.

- Obtain common signs and symptoms of a UTI from any textbook or reference book: decreased output, foul odor, dark color, dysuria, frequency, tenderness over urinary bladder, elevated temperature.
- The client's symptoms are consistent with the textbook or reference description of a UTI. He is not experiencing dysuria or frequency, but he is experiencing low back pain, which could mean that the infection is spreading to his kidneys.

2. Why is the client at increased risk for the development of a UTI?
   a. Define unknown terms such as dysuria, retention, and so forth.
   b. Review factors commonly associated with UTIs in a textbook or reference book.
      - UTIs are commonly associated with indwelling urinary catheters, urinary retention, inadequate fluid intake, decreased mobility, advanced age, and so on.
   c. Compare those factors with the data available about the client.
      - The client has many of the factors that place him at risk for a UTI, such as decreased mobility, inadequate fluid intake, presence of indwelling catheter, possibly inadequate perineal care, the aging process, and so forth.

3. Are there errors in your conclusions about the care provided by the client's wife?
   a. Identify conclusions you drew about the care provided by the client's wife (there are many possibilities).
      - The client's wife is doing the best she can. She does not have enough information to understand what is taking place. She is not physically capable of caring for her husband, who is difficult to care for, and so forth.
   b. Consider your conclusions. Is there a possibility any of them are wrong?
      - The conclusions could be wrong. There is not enough data to make any conclusions about the care the client's wife is providing or is capable of providing.

4. What attitude and cognitive critical thinking components did you use to answer the questions pertaining to this case?

   a. Question #1 requires divergent thinking.
      - Distinguishing relevant from irrelevant data
      - Clustering data into related patterns based on relevance

   b. Question #2 requires clarification.
      - Defining terms (urinary retention, dysuria)
      - Comparing the classic clinical manifestations of UTI with the client's clinical manifestations

   c. Question #3 requires intellectual integrity.
      - Admitting there are errors in the conclusions you drew

Preface to the Instructor's Edition

Unique to this *Instructor's Annotated Edition* is a set of student activity suggestions focusing on how students can answer the critical thinking questions. The suggestions are highlighted in **bold** and appear underneath each question. *Keep in mind that critical thinking questions do not always have one "right" answer, so you will receive a variety of answers from students.* It is most important that students are given the opportunity to provide rationale for their thinking and decision making.

The suggestions will help you give direction to students who may be having difficulty. For example, the question, "What conclusions can you draw about this client's heath status?" has several suggestions, such as "cluster data into related categories..." or "draw your conclusions based on health patterns you identify..." Another way to use the suggested student activities is to direct students to perform those tasks as a means of answering the question. For example, for the question, "How would you feel if you were in this client's situation?" you might want to tell the students, "Think about both your positive and negative feelings and identify how you might feel in this situation."

Occasionally you will see a reference to NIC or NOC in the suggested student activities. These acronyms refer to Nursing Interventions Classification (NIC) and Nursing Outcomes Classification (NOC), current nursing language classification systems being used by many nurses, nurse educators, and patient care facilities. More information about these classifications can be found in the following texts:

Marion Johnson & Meridean Maas. *Nursing Outcomes Classification* (NOC). Mosby Publishing Co. 1997.

Joanne McCloskey & Gloria Bulechek. *Nursing Interventions Classification (NIC)*, Mosby Publishing Co. 1996.

The last question posed in each case, "What attitude and cognitive critical thinking components did you use to address this case?" is particularly beneficial in that it urges students to consider their own thinking processes. You can direct students to think about and identify each of the critical thinking components they used based on content at the beginning of the workbook. You will be surprised at how rapidly students learn to identify critical thinking processes. The *Instructor's Annotated Edition* lists many of the critical thinking components required for each case, but other components are also possible.

You can assign a particular case to be discussed at the end of a classroom session or following a clinical day, and you can select one, two, or all of the questions based on your preference. Or, you may want to ask questions other than those listed. For example, you may want to use the case on *congestive heart failure*, but you want a greater emphasis placed on nursing interventions, patient outcomes, or pathophysiology. Simply add those questions when you assign the case. You may even want to use the case, but devise your own questions. Keep in mind, however, that the questions supplied are based on critical thinking theory and they are known to foster critical thinking.

Detailed Table of Contents

Introduction
Critical Thinking in Nursing

The complex legal, educational, and professional problems confronting nurses today emphasize the need for more than rote memory, knowledge of skills, and the ability to follow directions. Indeed, today critical thinking is an expected competency of nurses at all levels of education and practice. But you may be asking, "What is critical thinking, and how do I learn to think critically if I'm not doing so already?" This book is designed to answer that question. In the next few paragraphs you will be introduced to the concept of critical thinking and its common characteristics— characteristics that, when used, will become habit and will enhance your ability to think critically. Later in the book you will be given opportunities to practice using each of the skills introduced in this chapter.

Historical Perspective

Florence Nightingale is generally credited as the founder of modern nursing. There is evidence that Nightingale subscribed to methods of teaching that required critical thinking. Her students were required to keep case books in which they recorded, analyzed, and reflected upon activities on the ward. She regarded these diaries as useful because they required higher-order thinking and superior powers of observation (Seymer, 1960).

Nightingale emphasized the need for analytical skill development, however, nursing schools and instructors in the United States did little to foster thinking skills until the late 1800s. In 1898 an American nurse named Adelaide Nutting published an analysis of nurse training in the United States. She reported that nursing schools were doing little, if anything, to train the minds of students to observe, think, or reason accurately (Committee on Historical Materials, 1963). Nutting's report had an impact on the nursing community. By 1913, 20 states had enacted laws and regulations setting forth minimum requirements for nursing practice and education that included criteria related to thinking and decision making (Bixler, 1954; NLN, 1963).

During the 1920s, the lecture was the primary method used to teach nursing students. However, some nurse educators advocated the use of discussions, written assignments, and time for thinking (Henderson, 1982). Although these activities were limited primarily to ethical situations, they did require students to think about, not just memorize, the material. The concepts of thinking and problem solving were also introduced. In a handbook for nursing students, Jensen (1929) describes a method to analyze the patient's admission, care while hospitalized, and discharge. Perhaps Jensen's handbook served as the prototype for today's nursing process.

In 1927 the National League for Nursing Education (NLNE) published a revised *Curriculum Guide* for nursing schools that outlined important characteristics for nursing students. Good judgment, keen insight, use of discrimination, and the ability to detect physical and mental changes, draw conclusions, and make applications to other situations were some of those identified characteristics (NLN, 1927). The NLN *Curriculum Guide* revisions of 1937 and 1942 placed even greater emphasis on critical inquiry, independent thinking, good judgment, and resourcefulness (NLN, 1937, 1942). These characteristics are accepted today as components of critical thinking.

Despite the emphasis placed on thinking by nursing leaders of the '20s, '30s, and '40s, it was not until the late 1950s that a change in curricular structure actually took place. In 1953 Louise McManas proposed a set of functions unique to the professional nurse, today known as the nursing process and nursing diagnosis (McManas, 1953). McManas maintained that nurses who were taught the nursing process could be assumed to possess the ability to think reflectively and use higher analytical skills such as reasoning, judging, and drawing inferences. Today this assumption is highly debated. Many assert that the teaching nursing process is not, by itself, enough to produce critical thinkers.

Nurse educators and administrators in the 1960s began to turn their attention toward critical thinking and the use of critical thinking terminology (Gortner, 1977). The first report supporting the need for critical thinking concepts in nursing education was published in 1961 by the Institute of Research, part of the Teachers College of Columbia University. By 1963 an article appeared in the *Journal of Nursing Education* that clearly reflected the thinking of the period. It emphasized the importance of providing students with experiences that would encourage their development of critical thinking skills (Barbus, 1963). Even so, the '60s, '70s, and '80s found few educators calling for critical thinking; widespread acceptance and implementation was lacking.

Most recently, NLN representatives have begun to promote the use of activities that foster student thinking abilities. This move follows the national trend of the '80s to promote critical thinking at all levels of education. The NLN's most recent accreditation standards require nursing schools to provide evidence of student achievement of critical thinking. The need to include critical thinking in the nursing school curriculum is no longer an issue. Nutting's vision is now reality.

What Is Critical Thinking?

Critical thinking has as many definitions as there are authors writing about it. However, the following definitions are the most prevalent in critical thinking literature:

1. Critical thinking is reflective and reasonable thinking that is focused on what to believe or do (Ennis, 1985).

2. Critical thinking is an attitude of inquiry involving the use of principles, abstractions, deductions, interpretations, and analysis of arguments (Mathews, 1979).

3. Critical thinking is disciplined, self-directed thinking that exemplifies the perfections of thinking and displays mastery of intellectual skills and abilities; it is the art of thinking about your thinking while thinking in order to make your thinking better (Paul, 1990).

4. Critical thinking is an investigation whose purpose is to explore a situation, phenomenon, question, or problem to arrive at a hypothesis or conclusion about it that integrates all available information and can, therefore, be convincingly justified (Kurfiss, 1988).

5. Critical thinking is a rational investigation of ideas, inferences, assumptions, principles, arguments, conclusions, issues, statements, beliefs, and actions that covers scientific reasoning and includes the nursing process, decision making, and reasoning in controversial issues (Bandman & Bandman, 1995).

Critical thinking is a complex process that cannot be explained with a single definition. It is more important to familiarize yourself with the characteristics of critical thinking and to develop critical thinking habits. The purposes of this book and its activities are to acquaint you with the skills and attitudes associated with critical thinking and to provide you with practice opportunities for using the skills in your nursing courses.

Critical Thinking Attitudes

Critical thinking includes *attitudes* as well as cognitive skills. Robert Ennis (1985) referred to critical thinking attitudes as "dispositions." Richard Paul (1990) referred to them as "traits of mind." These attitudes motivate and justify the use of cognitive skills. Attitudes place the thinker in the right frame of mind for thinking. A critical thinker, as opposed to an ordinary thinker, will use one or more affective attitudes when thinking about what to believe or how to perform. Once you have engaged in exercises that focus your attention on attitudes, you will become aware of how often your thinking is affected by them. Seven interdependent attitudes or dispositions that are essential for becoming a critical thinker (Paul, 1990) are shown in the accompanying box and described in detail on the following page.

Intellectual Humility

Intellectual humility involves knowing and accepting the limits of your own knowledge.

> **Affective Attitudes of Critical Thinking**
>
> - Intellectual humility
> - Intellectual courage
> - Intellectual empathy
> - Intellectual integrity
> - Intellectual perseverance
> - Faith in reason
> - Intellectual sense of justice

Obviously, no one can know everything. What sets critical thinkers apart is that they understand the limits of their knowledge and recognize when they need to seek more information. For example, nurses who are critical thinkers and don't know anything about renal dialysis would consult an expert dialysis nurse before offering advice or actually performing the procedure.

Humility also involves being sensitive to your own prejudices or biases. A person who is prejudiced or biased has an opinion for or against something without having an adequate basis for that opinion. Nurses who are prejudiced against people with aquired immunodeficiency syndrome (AIDS) cannot always avoid caring for such clients. You might assume, then, that the care such nurses render to clients with AIDS would not be as good as that delivered to other clients. This assumption is incorrect. It is highly possible to deliver good care to people for whom we have negative opinions if we are aware of our prejudices and do not allow them to interfere with our judgments. As

another example, you may have a bias against a client with chronic obstructive pulmonary disease (COPD) who continues to smoke. As a critical thinker, you will recognize and acknowledge the bias without allowing it to negatively affect the care you render to the client. The following questions foster the development of the attitude of intellectual humility:

- How do your biases or prejudices affect the outcome of your client's care?
- What is your first impression of the client or client's situation?
- How will you know when you need more information?

Intellectual Courage

Intellectual courage involves the willingness to listen to and fairly evaluate the ideas, viewpoints, and beliefs of others even though you may not agree with these ideas or beliefs. Let's say that you feel strongly that the computerized documentation system that is being introduced at work (or school) will add to your workload instead of making your job easier. As a critical thinker, you will willingly listen to others who have a different perspective of computer documentation and base your judgment on what you *learn* rather than on just what you *feel*. In the end you may say, "Wow, I didn't realize that I will have the ability to access so much data by using this computer system. This may work after all!"

Examples of exercises that will allow you to practice and develop intellectual courage include the following:

- Explain how you feel about any topic to which you have a strong aversion, repugnance, or dislike.
- Defend the opposite point of view. For example, argue from the family's perspective in favor of placing a client on life support even though the degree of brain damage he has suffered may leave him unable to function with any degree of independence.

Intellectual Empathy

Intellectual empathy necessitates imagining yourself in the place of another in order to fully understand that other. For example, by imagining yourself in the place of a client who has just been told he has cancer, you will be better able to understand why he chooses to either undergo or refuse chemotherapy. Developing intellectual empathy may be readily accomplished by answering the following questions:

- Imagine that you have AIDS. Your nurses have been avoiding your room and you are quite sure that they do not want to care for you. How do you feel?
- You are in pain but no one has answered the call light. What are you thinking right now?
- You are awaiting the arrival of your home health nurse who is now 2 hours late. How does that make you feel?

Intellectual Integrity

When you hold your own evidence to the same standard of proof to which you hold others, you are demonstrating intellectual integrity. For example, when you read the results of research studies, you want to know how and why the researchers drew their conclusions. Were their instruments valid and reliable? What proof do they offer that their findings are accurate? Critical thinkers would apply the same test of proof to their own thinking: Are my assumptions based on data that are present? Are my conclusions accurate? How do I know that my thinking is "good"? Intellectual integrity can be developed by performing the following exercises:

- Make an argument in favor of something that you do not believe in or support.
- Ask yourself, "Do I use the same criteria to argue for this issue as I would to argue for something that I believe in?"
- Address situations like this one: Your employer has proposed 12-hour shifts, and you have proposed 10-hour shifts. Design criteria to equally evaluate both proposals.

Intellectual Perseverance

Intellectual perseverance is similar to other forms of perseverance. For example, nursing school can be difficult at times, but you are willing to persevere through the frustrations and difficulties because you know that your hard work will pay big dividends in the future. As a critical thinker, when you strive for the truth or for better understanding in spite of repeated frustrations and difficulties because you feel it is worth the effort in the long run, you are using the skill of intellectual perseverance. Projects that enforce or test intellectual perseverance may have the following qualities:

- A high degree of difficulty and requiring a long time to complete, such as collecting data about the functions of all community agencies in your area and the populations they serve.
- Multiple dimensions or a difficult problem that has no one "right" answer or solution, such as removing a person from mechanical life or nutritional support.

Faith in Reason

Faith in reason means believing that it is in the best interest of humankind for every person to develop the best possible thinking skills. The critical thinker supports this assumption and believes that all people can learn to think and reason critically. When your nursing faculty members encourage you to draw your own conclusions and develop your rational thinking skills, they are demonstrating the trait of faith in reason. They understand that it is in the best interest of all when nursing students learn to think independently and effectively. This skill may be developed by answering the following questions:

- What are the advantages and disadvantages of thinking this problem through before making a decision?
- What are the possible consequences if you do not use good thinking skills when planning or delivering care?

Intellectual Sense of Justice

This trait implies that, as a critical thinker, you will assess all viewpoints similarly without regard to vested interests or feelings or the vested interests or feelings of friends, community, or nation. For example, you may be discussing a new piece of equipment with a friend and several other colleagues. Your intellectual sense of justice will allow you to listen to everyone's viewpoints about the equipment and weigh them equally without showing preference toward your friend's opinion.

You can develop an intellectual sense of justice by solving problems such as this one: Despite your belief that individuals are responsible for the decisions they make or have made in the past, argue in favor of the lifelong smoker who should receive the same medical insurance coverage as you receive, even if he develops lung cancer as a result of his cigarette smoking.

You might have noticed that the affective attitudes of critical thinking are *interdependent* and *relevant* to all domains of knowledge. The definitions of such attitudes often overlap, and each of the suggested activities may enhance others. The greater your awareness of these attitudes or traits of mind, the better you will become at using them (Paul, 1990).

Critical Thinking Skills

The cognitive components of critical thinking are referred to as *abilities* or *skills* that an individual may or may not choose to use.

> **Cognitive Skills of Critical Thinking**
>
> • Divergent thinking
>
> • Reasoning
>
> • Reflection
>
> • Creativity
>
> • Clarification
>
> • Basic Support

Unlike the definition of critical thinking, there is general agreement about many cognitive components of critical thinking (see the accompanying box).

Divergent Thinking

One of the most prevalent cognitive components of critical thinking is divergent thinking. This is the ability of an individual to analyze a diversity of opinions and judgments (Perry, 1978). When practicing nurses obtain histories from their clients, they must separate out all irrelevant data, analyze pertinent data, and explore possibilities in order to draw accurate conclusions. When they follow this process, they are using the cognitive skill of divergent thinking. This skill can be developed through activities such as distinguishing relevant from irrelevant data, drawing accurate inferences, analyzing arguments, and recognizing the strengths or limitations of opposing viewpoints (Paul, 1990; White, 1990). Relevant data is generally thought of as abnormal data, whereas irrelevant data is nice to know but will not alter the person's care. An *inference* is a conclusion or deduc-

tion drawn about data, and *analyzing* means to closely study or evaluate data. Specific questions that enhance divergent thinking may include the following:

- Of the above data, which are most relevant to your care of this client?
- How do you know if this drug is effective? Ineffective?
- How will the care of this client with COPD help you care for your client with congestive heart failure?
- What can be inferred about this group of data?

Reasoning

Reasoning involves the general principles of logic. Critical thinkers should be able to discriminate between observation and inference, between fact (truth) and conjecture (guess or belief), and draw conclusions for themselves. Two types of reasoning are essential to critical thinking—inductive and deductive. *Inductive reasoning* involves generalization. For example, when you note that your client with advanced COPD experiences fatigue with activity and conclude that all clients with advanced lung disorders may experience fatigue with activity, you are using inductive reasoning. You use *deductive reasoning* when you draw conclusions about individuals on the basis of observations from a larger group. For example, you know that all postoperative clients are at increased risk for pain; therefore, you assume that your client who has just undergone hip surgery will most likely experience pain.

Questions that allow you to practice the cognitive skill of reasoning may include the following:

- Which data best support your conclusions?
- What process did you use to derive your conclusions?

Reflection

Reflection means to ponder, contemplate, or deliberate something. It takes time and cannot be done during an emergency. Reflection entails the ability to recognize that critical thinking is a multidimensional, rather than a linear or step-by-step, process. Critical thinkers are free to integrate new ideas or insights at any time or change their opinions when new evidence has been presented. Reflective thinking integrates past experiences into the present and explores potential alternatives. It involves drawing contingency-related, or "if . . . then", conclusions. For example, you may draw on your past experiences in caring for a sick child when planning care for a pediatric client. Or you may conclude that *if* you finish reading this chapter now, *then* you will have time to go to a movie later. Specifically, the cognitive skill of reflection can be practiced by asking the following questions:

- *If* the client, who had dyspnea (shortness of breath) benefited from this intervention, *then* perhaps another client will benefit as well.
- What experiences from my past impact the care I deliver to this client today?

Creativity

Creative thinking enables you to produce ideas and alternatives, use problem-solving strategies, and consider multiple solutions. For example, when nurses call a group of peers together to plan more effective ways for dealing with a particularly problematic client, they are using creative thinking skills. Creative thinking also involves use of our intuitive inferences. Everyone has heard of nurses who contend that they had a "gut" feeling that something was wrong with their client and, upon further investigation, found out they were right. Critical thinkers pay attention to their intuitions and integrate their "feelings" into their thinking and decision making. Novice nurses should, however, be cautioned to check their gut feelings with experienced nurses before acting on them. The cognitive skill of creativity can be developed through the following activities:

- Exploring alternative solutions to a client's problem.
- Finding a new way of performing a task when equipment is not available.
- Proposing an alternative way of implementing care that will result in the same or a similar outcome but reduce cost or length of hospital stay.
- Answering the question, "What do I feel about this situation?"

Clarification

Clarification includes skills such as noting similarities and differences, identifying assumptions, and defining terms (Norris &

Ennis, 1989). Clarification is one of the easier components to understand. When you compare acute pain with chronic pain, you are looking for ways in which both types of pain are the same, as well as exploring their differences. Nurses need to know the definitions of terms if they are to accurately interpret their usage. For example, it is difficult to know what to do for a patient's dysuria if you do not know that it means burning upon urination.

Assumptions are based on beliefs you've never questioned and may not even know you have. For example, when you see people who are dirty and dressed in tattered clothing, do you automatically assume that they are homeless or poor? Or do you simply assume that people can be dirty for a variety of reasons and make no inferences about the person's appearance? Identifying our assumptions and recognizing how those assumptions can affect our thinking are important aspects of critical thinking. The cognitive skill of clarification is being used when you do the following:

- Compare and contrast one concept with another, such as hypersensitivity with immunodeficiency, or activity intolerance with altered activities of daily living.
- Note similarities and differences in a concept, disease, or nursing diagnosis.
- Identify your assumptions.
- Define terms.

Basic Support

Basic support involves the use of known facts and background knowledge. Facts are truths. For example, normal body temperature is 98.6F when taken orally. It is necessary to know what the normal body temperature is before we can engage in thinking about all the reasons why a person's temperature may not be normal. It is difficult or impossible to think critically about anything if we have little or no knowledge about that which we are thinking.

Basic support further involves making and judging our observations and the credibility of our sources of information (Norris & Ennis, 1989). For example, would you take the word of the nursing assistant over the word of the dietary aide regarding the client's intake? You might. It would depend on the circumstances and which person picked up the client's food tray. Or, do you give as much credibility to the *Reader's Digest* as you do to a nursing journal? Nurses use their background knowledge and known facts about all aspects of care daily when caring for others. When they do so, they are using the basic support component of critical thinking.

The following questions foster the development of basic support:

- Upon what facts are you basing your conclusions?
- What is the consensus among researchers about the best way to deal with this problem?
- How does your background knowledge affect your current decisions?

Becoming a Critical Thinker

Now that you have an understanding of critical thinking and its attitudes and skills, you are ready to begin thinking critically. Remember, you will have to practice using higher-order thinking skills until they become comfortable and automatic. The exercises in this book will require you to use a variety of critical thinking skills, as well as identify and think about the skills you are using. In this way, you will become familiar with higher-order thinking and develop a level of comfort with its use.

The critical thinking skills and attitudes presented in this chapter are not all-inclusive, but they represent the skills most commonly identified with critical thinking. They are interrelated and interdependent; thus, practicing one skill will help you develop others. As you learn more about critical thinking, you will most likely be able to identify other skills that can also be considered critical thinking skills.

Critical Thinking Practice Session

Session One

Answer the following questions:

- What is your social security number?
- How many days are in September?
- What is the normal body temperature?

1. What kind of answers do these questions require?

2. What kind of thinking did you use to answer these questions?

Session Two

You have been notified by your employer that the primary parking lot for your building will be inaccessible for the next few months. Parking spaces have been obtained about a half mile from work, and a shuttle bus will be available to transport employees from the satellite parking lot to your building about every 15 minutes. Your employer has strongly urged you to use the satellite parking. You realize that you will have to leave for work at least a half hour earlier each day in order to park in the satellite lot. Upon expressing your concern to a friend, she advises you to park wherever you wish as there is no specific policy indicating that you must park off-site.

1. What is your first reaction about where you should park?

2. What is your decision about where to park?

3. Who or what most influenced you to make the decision you made?

4. What critical thinking *attitudes* influenced your thinking?

5. What critical thinking *cognitive skills* did you use?

Session Three

A 42-year-old woman who is 5 ft 2 in tall has recently experienced a change in weight and now weighs 150 lbs. You note that she is wearing a loose-fitting, baggy sweat suit.

1. What conclusions can you make about this client?

2. Upon what assumptions did you base your conclusions?

3. What information (data) do you need to verify your conclusions?

4. What biases are apparent in this case?

5. What critical thinking *attitudes* influenced your thinking about the client?

6. What *cognitive skills* did you use when considering the client's appearance?

Possible Answers to Critical Thinking Practice Sessions

Session One

1. These answers are facts.

2. Memory, recall, and the cognitive skill of basic support.

Session Two

1. Several reactions are possible: follow your employer's guidelines and take the shuttle to work; ignore your employer's guidelines and park where you usually park; or consider parking in another area altogether.

2. No suggestions.

3. Possibilities: the need to follow directions; fear of consequences; duty to your employer; or a previous experience with a similar situation.

4. Possibilities: faith in reason and intellectual sense of justice.

5. Possibilities: divergent thinking, reflection, and reasoning.

Session Three

1. Many conclusions are possible, but none may be correct. For example, the client may have gained weight and is trying to conceal it (a biased conclusion); she may have lost a lot of weight but has recently gained a few pounds back; she may be pregnant; or she may just want to be comfortable. No accurate conclusions can be drawn on the basis of the information provided.

2. Possible assumptions: overweight people try to hide their weight (a biased assumption), or overweight people wear large clothes and tend to be sloppy (another biased assumption).

3. Data needed: what is her recent weight gain or weight loss; is she dressed for comfort, has she been exercising, or is she pregnant?

4. Biases depend on assumptions and beliefs. If you concluded that she was attempting to hide her weight, based on erroneous assumptions, then your bias is against overweight people.

5. Intellectual humility and intellectual empathy.

6. Possibilities: analysis, divergent thinking, and reflection.

References

Bandman, E., & Bandman, B. (1995). *Critical thinking in nursing* (2nd ed.) Norwalk, CT: Appleton & Lange.

Barbus, A., & Carbol, K. (1963). Experiences in problem-solving for the baccalaureate student. *The Journal of Nursing Education*, 11–20.

Bixler, R. & Bixler, G. (1954). *Administration for nursing education*. New York: G. P. Putnam's Sons.

Committee on Historical Source Materials in Nursing (1963). Three score years and ten, 1883–1963. New York: National League for Nursing.

Ennis, R. (1985). *A taxonomy of critical thinking dispositions and abilities*. Illinois Critical Thinking Project. University of Illinois, Champaign.

Gortner, S., & Nahm, H. (1977). An overview of nursing research in the United States. *Nursing research*, 26(1), 10–33.

Henderson, V. (1982). Nursing process–is the title right? *Journal Advances in Nursing*. Mar 7:103–109.

Jensen, D. (1929). *Nursing care studies*. (1st ed.) New York: The Macmillan Company.

Jensen, D. (1940). *Nursing care studies*. (3rd ed.) New York: The Macmillan Company.

Kurfiss, J. (1988). *Critical thinking: theory, research, practice, and possibilities*. ASHE-ERIC Higher Education Report No. 2. Washington, D.C.: Association for the Study of Higher Education, 2–3.

Mathews, C. (1979). Nursing diagnoses from the perspective of concept attainment and critical thinking. *Advances in Nursing Science*, 2, 17–26.

McManas, L. (1953). Assumptions and functions of nursing. In *Regional planning for nursing and nursing education*: Report of work conference held by the division of nursing education. New York: Teachers College, Columbia University.

National League for Nursing Education (1927). *A curriculum guide for schools of nursing*, New York.

National League for Nursing Education (1937). *A curriculum guide for schools of nursing,* (2nd ed.), New York.

National League for Nursing (1942). *Essentials of a good school of nursing*, New York.

National League for Nursing (1963). *Three score years and ten, 1883–1963*, New York.

Norris, S., & Ennis, R. (1989). *Evaluating critical thinking*. Pacific Grove, California: Critical Thinking Press and Software.

Perry, W. (1978). Growth in making of meaning: Youth into adulthood. In A. Chickering (Ed.) *The future of american colleges*. San Francisco: Jossey-Bass.

Paul, R. (1990). *Critical thinking*. Rohnert Park, CA: The Center for Critical Thinking and Moral Critique, Sonoma State University.

Seymer, L. R. (1960). One hundred years ago. *American Journal of Nursing*. May, 658–661.

White, N., Beardslee, N., Peters, D., & Supples, J. (1990). Promoting critical thinking skills. *Nurse Educator*, 15(5), 16-19.

Adult Health Nursing

Adult Health Nursing
Abdominal Aortic Aneurysm

The client is a 65-year-old retired farmer who lives on a 200-acre farm with his wife of 45 years. He has three grown sons who live in nearby communities. He enjoyed good health until about 7 years ago when he was placed on antihypertensive medications to control his blood pressure. He is 5 ft, 9 in tall and weighs 258 lbs. His physician has repeatedly expressed concern about his weight, but the client enjoys eating and has been unsuccessful in controlling his weight since his retirement.

Earlier today, the client began experiencing moderate to severe abdominal pain. Unable to reach their primary care provider by telephone, the client's wife drove her husband to the emergency department. The nurse there noted a large, pulsating mass in the client's upper abdomen. She assessed his vital signs and immediately notified the physician of her findings. Radiologic examination confirmed the presence of an abdominal aortic aneurysm. In light of the client's clinical presentation, the physician contacted a surgeon who recommended immediate surgical intervention.

~~~~

1. What are the client's priority nursing diagnoses at this time?

   - Discuss the implications of emergency surgery versus elective surgery.

   - Consider the client's emotional needs as well as his physical needs.

   - Identify essential monitoring that must be done in order to detect leakage of the aneurysm while the client is awaiting surgery.

   - Identify appropriate nursing diagnoses on the basis of the client's data. Prioritize the nursing diagnoses, noting whether physical or emotional concerns take precedence.

2. What is the relationship between the client's abdominal aneurysm, his hypertension, and the need for emergency surgery?

   - Review the pathophysiology of and contributing factors to abdominal aortic aneurysms.

   - Discuss the impact of increased blood pressure on an aneurysm and the dangers of leakage or rupture.

   - Speculate about the consequences of not doing the surgery.

3. What could have occurred if the nurse had not used critical thinking skills when assessing the client?

   - Discuss the complications associated with a leaking abdominal aortic aneurysm, such as hypovolemic shock or death.

   - Discuss the need for correlating the patient's medical history with current clinical manifestations.

   - Discuss the consequences of inadequate assessment and data collection.

4. What risks are involved in performing surgery on the client?

   Review factors that increase a person's risk for complications during and after a surgical procedure. Consider, for example, age, weight, physical status, and chronic disease. Speculate about how each of these factors increase the risk for complications such as atelectasis, wound healing, bleeding, and so on.

5. What have you learned about this case that may guide your care of other emergency surgery patients with different medical diagnoses?

   - Consider the spectrum of clients who must undergo emergency surgery such as ectopic pregnancy, ruptured appendix, and coronary bypass. Compare their emotional and physical needs with those of the client.

   - Consider the impact of obesity on respiratory status, healing, and handling by operating room personnel, regardless of the type of surgery.

   - Consider the impact of hypertension and the need for close monitoring and blood pressure control during and after surgery.

6. What critical thinking components did you use to address this case?

   Divergent thinking, creativity, reasoning, faith in reason, among others.

Adult Health Nursing
Acute Lymphocytic Leukemia

The client is a 62-year-old retired school teacher and mother of three children, all of whom are married and live more than 100 miles away. Her youngest daughter has temporarily moved back home to assist her mother. The client's husband is supportive but is often emotionally distraught and tearful.

Two months ago, the client began experiencing extreme weakness and fatigue. Prior to that, she had tired easily, experienced difficulty recovering from a cold, and noticed a wound on her left ankle that failed to heal. She also experienced slight bleeding of her gums when brushing her teeth, as well as decreased appetite. By the time she consulted her physician, she had lost 10 lbs and was running a fever of 100F. Her physician conducted blood studies and a bone marrow aspiration, which led to the diagnosis of acute lymphocytic leukemia. Currently, the client is hospitalized, has a Groshong catheter in place, and is undergoing a regimen of chemotherapy drugs, including vincristine, prednisone, and methotrexate.

Consultations by the social worker resulted in the following notations: Client has been tearful on the last two visits. She states, "I'm just so tired of being sick. I'm not sure that I can go through any more chemotherapy. My husband is so dependent on me. He keeps pushing me to fight this disease. My daughter thinks I should try imagery and nutritional supplements. I don't want to die yet, but I don't think I have any fight left in me. I'm not afraid of dying."

The client has been a diabetic since the age of 25. She takes 10 units of regular insulin at breakfast and 30 units of NPH insulin at bedtime. She has undergone no major surgeries other than a tonsillectomy at age 5. She has no known allergies.

Upon examination, the client is oriented to person, time, and place. Her grips are equal. She complains of headache and dizziness upon standing and slight numbness and tingling of her lower extremities. Petechiae cover her arms, chest, and upper thighs. Her skin is pale, with diminished turgor, and her oral mucous membranes are dry. There is a small ulcerated area on the outer aspect of her left ankle. Her Groshong site is clean and dry but slightly red. Her apical heart rate is 90 beats per minute (bpm) and regular. Her pedal pulses are 1+ bilaterally, and her extremities are cool to touch. Her blood pressure is 140/84 lying and 128/72 standing. Her respirations are 20 breaths per minute and regular. She has no obvious dyspnea but complains of shortness of breath upon exertion. Her lung sounds are clear in all fields. Her sputum is slightly yellow in color. Her abdomen is soft with bowel sounds present in all four quadrants; she denies pain or tenderness with palpation.

The client's diagnostic findings include the following:

Hematology: WBC 9000, RBC 2.23, Hgb 8.8 g/dL, Hct 26%, platelets 12,000/mm^3

CBC differential: neutrophils serum 10%, bands 1%, lymphocytes 60%

Chemistry profile: glucose 250 mg/dL, albumin 2.4 g/dL, Ca 8.0 mEq/L

~~~~

1. What are the client's most important nursing diagnoses and why did you prioritize them the way you did?

   - Group data into physiologic and emotional problems, for example, physical: fatigue, wound that will not heal, risk for infection related to Groshong catheter and/or diabetes, and immunosuppression related to chemotherapy; emotional: client is tired of being sick, husband is dependent and depressed, and daughter is pressing client to use alternative therapies.

   - Prioritize problems on the basis of life-preservation criteria or Maslow's hierarchy of needs. Discuss your reasons for prioritizing according to that criteria.

2. What is the relationship between the client's absolute granulocyte count (AGC) and her risk for infection?

   - Calculate the client's AGC (white blood cells [WBCs] x neutrophils + bands = AGC [900 x .11 = 99]). Review the function of granulocytes and discuss the consequences of reduced cell numbers on immune competence.

   - Discuss the risks of infection posed from immunosuppression and all possible sources of infection, for example, catheter-insertion site, nonhealing wound, and diabetes.

3. How will you know if the client is developing an infection?

   - Review the signs and symptoms that commonly denote a beginning local or systemic infection in the immunocompromised host.

   - Discuss the assessment parameters designed to detect infections, such as fever or chills, redness, or swelling at the wound or catheter-insertion site.

   - Discuss how infections differ in the immunocompromised host.

4. How can you best intervene to assist the client at this time?

   - Discuss the use of the Nursing Interventions Classification (NIC) to assist the nurse in planning care for the client.

   - Review the problems identified in question 1 and select interventions most appropriate for those problems.

   - List nursing interventions that address decision making, anxiety reduction, coping enhancement, family-process maintenance, family support, prevention of infection, fatigue, fluid and electrolyte maintenance, and so on.

5. What can you do to ease the effects of chemotherapy for the client?

   - Research the medications that the client is using to determine side effects commonly associated with the drugs. Identify nursing activities commonly used to prevent, reduce, or relieve medication side effects.

   - Explore alternative methods of relieving anxiety, nausea, vomiting, or other symptoms associated with chemotherapy, such as distraction or massage.

6. What impact may the client's diabetes have on her leukemia?

   • Discuss conditions commonly associated with diabetes, such as decreased circulation, slowed healing, and so on.

   • Explore the potentiating effect of one disease on another.

   • Identify signs and symptoms of leukemia that may be worsened by diabetes.

7. How will you prepare the client for discharge from the hospital?

   • Discuss care that will be needed when the client goes home, such as nutritional support; household assistance; the ability to perform her own activities of daily living (ADLs), comply with medical treatment protocols, and offer support to her husband; the ability of her family to be involved in her care, and so on.

   • Identify important teaching, community referrals, and respite care.

8. What critical thinking components did you use to answer the questions pertaining to this case?

   Divergent thinking, reasoning, clarification, intellectual empathy, among others.

Adult Health Nursing
Acute Pulmonary Edema

The client is a 59-year-old man admitted to the emergency department with complaints of severe shortness of breath and a cough producing frothy, blood-tinged mucous. His history reveals a myocardial infarction 2 years ago. Since then, he has been on a low-salt diet, digoxin, and furosemide for control of congestive heart failure.

The client is admitted to the hospital for treatment of acute pulmonary edema secondary to congestive heart failure. On his fourth hospital day, the client complains of tingling and numbness of his fingers, muscle weakness, and palpitations. His electrocardiogram shows frequent premature ventricular contractions (PVCs). Four hours later, he is confused and restless.

The client's diagnostic findings are as follows:

Arterial blood gases: pH 7.55, $PaCO_2$ 25 mm Hg, HCO_3 34 mEq/L, PaO_2 65 mm Hg, SaO_2 91%

Hematology: K 2.5 mEq/L

~~~~

1. What conclusions can you draw about the client's clinical manifestations, PaO_2, and SaO_2 levels?

   - Analyze clinical manifestations, noting those that are reflective of oxygenation.

   - Review normal findings for PaO_2 and SaO_2 and compare them with the client's levels.

   - Discuss the concepts of hypoxia and hypoxemia.

   - List possible problems related to the client's present state of oxygenation. Consider hypoxia, acid-base imbalance, and so on.

2. What are the most likely causes of the client's acid-base imbalance?

   * Review the concepts of acid-base balance and imbalance, respiratory compensation, and metabolic compensation. On the basis of the data provided, interpret the client's blood gases.

   * Investigate common factors that contribute to the development of acid-base imbalance and compare those factors with the client's data.

   * Identify the most likely cause of the client's acid-base imbalance.

3. What is the relationship between the client's arterial blood gas values and his serum potassium level?

   * Review factors that negatively alter serum potassium levels. Review the effects of acid-base imbalance on serum potassium levels.

   * Discuss the significance of a serum potassium of 2.5 mEq/L.

   * Identify possible consequences to the client if his hypokalemia is not addressed.

4. What are the priority nursing diagnoses for the client?

   Group objective and subjective data into problem categories. Prioritize problems into those that need to be addressed immediately versus those that can wait. Use Maslow's hierarchy of needs, life preservation, or other criteria to establish priorities.

5. What nursing actions can be implemented to address the client's priority nursing diagnoses?

   * Discuss the client's anxiety, hypokalemia and associated PVCs, acid-base imbalance, hypoxia, and so on.

   * Consider interventions to control or reduce his anxiety; prevent, monitor, or report abnormal electrolytes or acid-base imbalances; reduce or eliminate hypoxia, and so forth.

   * Investigate the Nursing Interventions Classification (NIC) for interventions specific to acid-base imbalance, hypokalemia, or hypoxia.

6. What critical thinking components did you use to address this case?

   Divergent thinking, clarification, faith in reason, intellectual empathy, among others.

Adult Health Nursing
Adenocarcinoma of the Colon

The client is a 47-year-old father of eight children, ranging in ages from 7 to 22. Five children are still living at home. His children and wife are supportive and concerned. Six months ago, the patient sought medical attention after several months of abdominal discomfort, which included alternating constipation and diarrhea. A colonoscopy revealed a large tumor of the sigmoid colon. The diagnosis of widespread adenocarcinoma of the colon with metastasis to the liver was confirmed by exploratory surgery.

The client has been admitted to the hospital for severe, intractable abdominal and back pain. He does not want to be too sedated but states that he can no longer stand the pain. The client's appetite has diminished, and he has lost approximately 12 lbs in approximately 1 month. He and his wife are considering hospice care. In addition, his older daughter is concerned about her father's long-term use of narcotics.

The client's health history includes hypertension and early coronary artery disease. Home medications include 60 mg of oral morphine sulfate per day, 100 mg of Lopressor daily, and 80 mg of verapamil three times daily. The client is allergic to penicillin.

Upon examination, the client is sedate, oriented, and cooperative. His skin is slightly jaundiced, warm, and dry. His oral mucous membranes are moist and pink. His lungs are clear bilaterally, and his respiratory rate is 18 breaths per minute; he denies shortness of breath. His apical rate is 82 beats per minute (bpm) and irregular. He has 3+ peripheral edema and slight jugular vein distention, and his blood pressure is 170/90, which represents an increase from his usual blood pressure. His abdomen is somewhat firm with hyperactive bowel sounds, and his abdominal girth is 38 inches (increased from normal by 2 inches). He complains of anorexia, nausea, indigestion, constipation, and flatulence. His urine output over the past 8 hours was 600 mLs of dark brownish urine. He denies pain or burning on urination.

The client's diagnostic findings are as follows:

Hematology: WBC 6000, Hgb 9.9 g/dL, Hct 28%

Coagulation: prothrombin time 25 seconds

Chemistry profile: Indirect bilirubin 2.8 mg/dL, Serum albumin 2.5 mg/dL, SGPT 129 U/L, LDH 384 U/L, K 3.0 mEq/L, Na 129 mEq/L

~~~~

1. What inferences, can be made from the data provided about the client?

   • Review data and cluster into categories. Consider clustering data by body systems, health patterns, or groups that seem related.

   • Using data clusters, identify possible problems and priority nursing diagnoses.

   • Decide what inferences can be made from each data cluster, for example, the client's mental status, family support, his prognosis, his family's ability to cope with his illness or prognosis, his current physical problems, and the physical problems that he will have to face related to his chemotherapy.

2. In your opinion, do the client's emotional or physical problems take precedence?

   • Divide the clustered data into physical and psychosocial nursing diagnoses.

   • Consider which nursing diagnoses are more important to the client and to his family at this time. Speculate about how his prognosis may impact his physical care and his psychosocial care.

   • Imagine yourself in the client's situation. Would your physical or psychosocial needs take precedence?

3. What evidence suggests that the client is experiencing fluid overload?

   • Review the concept of fluid overload and the signs and symptoms suggestive of fluid overload.

   • Compare the expected assessment findings with the client's signs and symptoms.

   • Explore the relationships between fluid overload and hypertension, peripheral edema, and decreased urine output.

4. What interventions are most appropriate for the client at this time?

- Review priority data and select interventions pertinent to the identified problems.

- Consider interventions that address the client's chemotherapy management, his ability to cope with his treatments, fluid status, potential for infection, pain management, family support systems, and so on.

5. What other knowledge or information would be useful when planning care for the client?

Review all aspects of adenocarcinoma of the colon. Speculate about information that would be useful, such as current effective treatment protocols for cancer of the colon or liver, the potential for cure of metastatic cancer, whether the client is considering chemotherapy or other treatment possibilities, his need for spiritual assessment or intervention, and his and his family's outlook on death.

6. Why is liver metastasis an issue when planning medication therapies for pain management?

- Review current medication therapies designed for pain management. Investigate the side effects and route of elimination of each medication.

- Identify drugs that are highly effective in controlling pain but may be contraindicated for patients with liver disease.

- Consider whether the pain medication that the client currently uses is the most appropriate drug for him considering the liver involvement.

- Explore the use of other medications that could effectively reduce pain without producing further liver compromise or discomfort.

7. How can you assist this family to reduce the costs associated with the client's care without compromising his quality of care or effective pain management?

- Consider the costs of acute-care hospitalization, home care, and hospice care. Explore the benefits and limitations of each type of care.

- Consider community support services that may be available and the cost of each service.

- On the basis of the information gathered, what suggestions can be given to the family for reducing or maintaining costs?

8. How legitimate is the daughter's concern about the client's use of narcotic analgesics?

  - Investigate the treatment of acute and chronic pain.

  - Explore factors that contribute to narcotic addiction and how those factors apply to the client's situation.

  - Speculate about the source of the daughter's concern other than that of narcotic addiction, such as fear that he will not recover, denial that he is terminally ill, and so on.

  - Discuss the merit of preventing narcotic addiction in patients with terminal diseases.

9. What critical thinking components did you use to answer the questions pertaining to this case?

  Divergent thinking, creativity, intellectual humility, and basic support.

Adult Health Nursing

Atrial Dysrhythmia: Rapid Heart Rate

A 60-year-old woman with a history of arteriosclerotic heart disease (ASHD) and hypertension is brought in to the emergency department by ambulance. She is complaining of nausea, anorexia, and blurred vision. She is alert and oriented, although her daughter states that the client has had periods of confusion over the past several days. The client explains that she is currently under her physician's care for episodes of atrial fibrillation and atrial flutter that began about 1 week ago. Home medications include 0.125 mg of digoxin daily, as well as quinidine sulfate and Catapres.

The nurse starts the client on 4 liters of oxygen by nasal cannula and an intravenous (IV) infusion of lactated Ringer's solution at 100 mL per hour. Her cardiac monitor reveals an atrial fibrillation with a ventricular rate of 180 beats per minute (bpm). Her blood pressure is stable at 120/82.

The client has been placed on pulse oximetry, and a 12-lead ECG, portable chest x-ray, and serum digoxin level have been obtained. The emergency room physician is considering a brief trial of IV diazepam prior to attempting other treatments, such as cardioversion for the client's rapid heart rate.

~~~~

1. What conclusions can you draw about the client's health status?

   Analyze data for cues or patterns. Think about her clinical manifestations, her complaints, the medications she is currently taking, the effect of those medications on cardiac rhythm, and her cardiac status. Consider inadequate digitalization, digitalis toxicity, and so on.

2. What is the significance of the client's current blood pressure of 120/82?

- Review accepted parameters for normal blood pressure, hypertension, and hypotension.

- Consider the client's history of hypertension.

- Conclude whether she is experiencing hypotension. Identify data that are necessary to confirm that she is hypotensive.

3. What are the possible outcomes if you administer diazepam at this time?

- Investigate the medication diazepam, noting its intended actions as well as its side effects. Consider the effect it may have on both heart rate and rhythm.

- Identify contraindications for the use of this drug, such as hypotension. Discuss the potentiating effects of diazepam on the client's hypotensive state.

4. What are the possible positive or negative effects of using digoxin for the client's atrial dysrhythmia?

- Investigate the medication digoxin, noting its intended benefits and identifying possible detrimental effects.

- Discuss the implications of administering more digoxin if the client is experiencing digitalis toxicity. Identify the expected drug effect if she is not experiencing digitalis toxicity.

- Discuss the clinical manifestations of digitalis toxicity and identify the laboratory values that support its presence.

5. What critical thinking components did you use to address this case?

Basic support, divergent thinking, reasoning, reflection, among others.

Adult Health Nursing

Bleeding Esophageal Varices

The client is a 68-year-old man with a history of chronic alcohol abuse. Five years ago, he was diagnosed with cirrhosis of the liver. His wife reports that he recently developed bronchitis accompanied by a persistent cough. He has been admitted to the emergency department with hematemesis and confusion. Currently, the client is complaining of severe thirst and dizziness. His skin and sclera appear mildly jaundiced.

The nurse practitioner in the emergency department notes an enlarged spleen and, upon rectal examination, notes the presence of hemorrhoids.

The client's diagnostic findings are as follows:

Hemotology: 8.0 g/dL, Hct 20%

Coagulation: prolonged prothrombin time

Chemistry profile: elevated total bilirubin, decreased albumin, and elevated ammonia

The nurse practitioner summons the emergency department physician and prepares the client for the insertion of a Sengstaken-Blakemore tube.

~~~~

1. What factors indicate the use of a Sengstaken-Blakemore tube for the client's problem?

   - Investigate the purpose and general use of the Sengstaken-Blakemore tube.

   - Speculate about the client's medical diagnosis on the basis of the need for this tube. Consider his history of cirrhosis, his history of bronchitis and coughing, and his potential for bleeding and subsequent hypovolemic shock.

2. How are cirrhosis of the liver and esophageal varices related?

- Review the pathophysiology and resulting consequences of alcohol abuse and liver cirrhosis.

- Discuss the buildup of ammonia from hepatic encephalopathy.

- Consider the causes of esophageal varices.

3. Which factors may have contributed to the development of esophageal varices and to the client's present problem?

Discuss risk factors that lead to the development of esophageal varices and the potential for their rupture and hemorrhage. Consider the inability of the liver to convert ammonia to urea for excretion, the large protein load from gastrointestinal bleeding that results in increased ammonia levels, hypoxia from blood loss, and so on. Consider the relationship between pressure created by coughing and the development of bleeding from esophageal varices.

4. What priority nursing actions are necessary to protect the client during and following insertion of the tube?

- Review the procedure for insertion of a Sengstaken-Blakemore tube and necessary monitoring during and after the procedure.

- Describe potential complications of tube insertion. Consider measures to prevent aspiration, the need for available suction equipment and scissors, the possibility of respiratory distress, and so on.

5. How could your biases about self-induced illness affect the care of the client?

- Identify biases that you may hold about patients who develop diseases related to their lifestyle habits.

- Identify other "socially unacceptable" diseases.

- Speculate about how biases may affect the care that patients receive.

- Discuss how you can provide quality care even if you do not agree with your clients' lifestyles.

6. What critical thinking components did you use to address this case?

Intellectual empathy, reasoning, creativity, basic support, and so on.

Adult Health Nursing
Breast Cancer

A 41-year-old divorced woman with four children, ages 7, 9, 12, and 15, sells real estate and is active in the community. Two weeks ago, upon routine mammography, a small but distinct lesion was noted in her left breast. She underwent a biopsy that was positive for ductal carcinoma. Consequently, her physician scheduled her for a lumpectomy.

The client has a history of deep vein thrombosis, originally related to taking birth control pills. Prior to this admission, her medication regimen consisted only of ASA. She is concerned about the outcome of the surgery and the prospect of undergoing chemotherapy or radiation. In fact, she has not made up her mind about undergoing chemotherapy. Her maternal aunt died of breast cancer after undergoing chemotherapy and the client is not convinced that chemotherapy will be effective in her case either. The client's parents live out of town but are supportive. Her mother is flying to town this evening to stay with the client's children during and immediately after her surgery.

The client is 5 ft, 5 in tall and weighs 138 lbs. Upon examination, she is alert and oriented. Her skin and mucous membranes are pink, intact, and moist. Her lungs are clear bilaterally with a respiratory rate of 18. Her heart rate is regular at 80 beats per minute (bpm). Her abdomen is soft and nontender, and bowel sounds are present in four quadrants. She has no extremity edema, and pedal pulses are strong and equal.

The client's diagnostic findings are as follows:

Chest x-ray: normal lung fields

Electrocardiogram: normal sinus rhythm, 82 bpm

Hematology: WBC 6,000; Hgb 11.9 g/dL, Hct 35%, RBC 3.9

Chemistry profile: glucose 109 mg/dL, albumin 3.8 g/dL, Ca 5.0 mg/dL, Cl 98 mEg/L, phosphorus 4.3 mg/dL, Mg 2.3 mg/dL, K 4.6 mEq/L

~~~~

1. What impact does the client's history of deep vein thrombosis have on her current situation?

   • Review the pathophysiology of deep vein thrombosis and factors that contribute to its development.

   • Review the risks that occur with any surgical procedure.

   • Discuss why patients with a previous history of deep vein thrombosis are at increased risk for future episodes, especially when undergoing surgery.

   • Collect information about birth control medications to find the relationship between the medication and development of deep vein thrombosis.

2. Given the client's medical history, current illness, and physical assessment, what are her priority nursing diagnoses?

   • Cluster data into physical and psychosocial problems.

   • Focus on her immediate need, which is preparation for surgery.

   • Discuss her potential for surgical complications, considering her history.

   • Discuss the appropriateness of nursing diagnoses such as anxiety, knowledge deficit, decisional conflict, treatment options, and so on. Prioritize these nursing diagnoses, providing rationale for the highest priority diagnoses.

3. What decisional conflict is the client experiencing?

   • Analyze the client's concerns, family situation, and medical history.

   • Discuss the impact of her aunt's death despite chemotherapy for breast cancer. Identify reasons why the client may not have the same outcome as her aunt. Identify reasons for trying every available treatment option.

   • Discuss how wanting to live conflicts with the feeling that treatments will not be effective.

4. Why is it unnecessary for the client to decide if she wants chemotherapy at this time, even though she has been diagnosed with ductal adenocarcinoma?

   • Discuss the need for staging of the tumor before treatment options such as chemotherapy can be discussed.

   • Review the TNM method of staging malignancies (T = size, depth, and extent of tumor growth; N = degree and location of lymph node involvement; M = presence or absence of metastasis).

   • Discuss the need to focus on the surgical procedure, its outcome, and the results of tumor staging prior to considering treatments or chemotherapy.

5. What nursing actions can you implement to address the client's priority nursing diagnoses?

   • Review the data obtained in question 1 and select the most appropriate interventions for the identified problems. Consider interventions that address decision making, reduction and control of anxiety, coping enhancement, family process maintenance, family support, and so on.

   • Discuss the use of the Nursing Interventions Classification (NIC) to assist the nurse in planning care for a client with cancer who is trying to make treatment decisions.

6. How may caring for the client help you plan care for a patient with aquired immunodeficiency syndrome (AIDS), chronic renal failure, or another chronic illness?

   • List characteristics that these client's have in common, such as a chronic illness that requires medical intervention, conflict regarding the pros and cons of treatment, feelings of hopelessness and helplessness, fear of being a burden to family members, and fear of dying.

   • Discuss the decisional conflicts that affect any client with a chronic illness.

   • Contemplate how a client's outlook is often influenced by the success or failure of another family member's treatment.

7. How may your personal biases affect your ability to advocate on behalf of the client if she chooses not to undergo chemotherapy?

- Examine your own biases about accepting or rejecting chemotherapy as a treatment option.

- Identify possible biases toward people who choose not to undergo conventional types of medical treatment even though they have a good chance of recovery. Consider that the lack of agreement with another's choice may make it difficult to advocate on his or her behalf.

- Discuss the need to identify your own biases in order to support people whose values are different from your own values.

8. What critical thinking components did you use to answer questions pertaining to this case?

Reasoning, reflection, clarification, intellectual sense of justice, among others.

Adult Health Nursing
Complicated Diabetes Mellitus

The client is a 63-year-old hair stylist who lives in a rural area with her retired husband and two dogs. She is the mother of two sons, both of whom live in other states but visit at least annually. The client plans to retire within the next year and is looking forward to pursuing her sewing and gardening hobbies on a full-time basis.

The client was diagnosed with type II (non-insulin-dependent) diabetes mellitus 5 years ago. She has maintained her diet and daily insulin injections with few difficulties until recently. Approximately 3 weeks ago she contracted influenza from one of her clients, which primarily manifested as a chronic productive cough and shortness of breath. Assuming that she would recover in a few days, the client stayed home from work but had difficulty eating or drinking due to loss of appetite and throat soreness related to coughing. At the insistence of her husband, she visited her family physician who subsequently admitted her to the hospital for pneumonia.

Currently, the client is receiving intravenous antibiotics and steroids, and her lungs are beginning to clear. Her cough is diminishing but remains productive.

Upon examination, the client is oriented to person and place but is lethargic and has difficulty answering your questions. When she does respond, she complains of nausea. Her skin is warm, dry, and flushed. Her pulse is 112 beats per minute (bpm), her blood pressure is 104/70, her oral temperature is 99.2F, and her respirations are 30 breaths per minute. Her intake and output record indicates that she has voided 850 mL of urine since 6:00 AM (it is now 10:00 AM), and she has taken in 700 mL of fluid. The glucometer indicates that her serum glucose is too high to register; therefore, it is at least 400 mg/dL.

The client's diagnostic findings are as follows:

Fasting glucose: 230 mg/dL

~~~~

1. What data are most relevant in determining priority nursing diagnoses for the client?

   Group data into physiological and psychosocial categories. Prioritize data groups according to Maslow's needs, life preservation criteria, or other prioritizing criteria. Identify the nursing diagnosis that is most appropriate for the data groups.

2. On the basis of the laboratory data and your assessment findings, what conclusions can you draw about the client?

   • Separate the client's data into normal and abnormal categories.

   • Discuss the clinical manifestations of hyperglycemia, hyperosmolar nonketotic coma (HNKC), and diabetic ketoacidosis (DKA).

   • Correlate the client's assessment data with common clinical manifestations of conditions that complicate type II diabetes mellitus.

   • Discuss serious risks from this condition such as fluid volume deficit.

3. What other data are essential in order to substantiate your suspicions?

   • Review diagnostic indicators for diabetes mellitus and its complications. Discuss the appropriateness of diagnostic tests for validating the presence or absence of complications.

   • Consider the client's last dose and type of insulin, the amount of food she ate at breakfast, and the nurse's response to her early morning fasting blood glucose.

4. What is the relationship between non-insulin-dependent diabetes mellitus (NIDDM) and (HNKC)?

- Review the pathophysiology of NIDDM as well as conditions and factors that may result in HNKC.

- Diagram the process of glucose alteration that results in HNKC, indicating normal and abnormal processes.

- Discuss the importance of regulating the blood sugar rapidly by treating the client with insulin, potassium, and sodium.

- Review the necessity of replacing potassium while lowering the blood sugar.

5. How would your assessment findings differ if the client was experiencing DKA?

- Review the pathophysiology of DKA and HNKC. List common assessment findings for each condition.

- Compare the client's assessment data with both conditions. Discuss how the client's assessment findings would have differed if she was experiencing DKA instead of HNKC.

- Speculate about the early symptoms of DKA versus late-onset symptoms.

6. What impact does the client's pneumonia have on her diabetes mellitus?

- Identify problems that can develop from pneumonia that may adversely affect diabetes mellitus, for example, decreased appetite or reduced intake with the same insulin dose; increased metabolic needs of the body when fighting an infection; and a reduction in normal activities, thus reducing the use of insulin, decreasing oxygenation, and minimizing the cells ability to function normally.

7. Why must you consider the client's current medications when evaluating her present situation?

   • Analyze the client's current medications. Decide if any of her medications are contributing to her increased blood glucose, for example, glucocorticoids are known to cause hyperglycemia.

   • Investigate common antibiotics, such as the penicillins and cephalosporins, to determine if they alter blood glucose levels.

8. To which other groups of patients can you generalize the care of the client?

   Consider other conditions that can result in hyperosmolar coma, such as clients receiving hyperalimentation, clients with severe burns, or clients undergoing renal dialysis. Compare these conditions to diabetes mellitus in regard to the pathophysiological changes they produce that result in HNKC. List clinical manifestations that will be similar for all clients experiencing this problem.

9. What critical thinking components did you use to answer the questions pertaining to this case?

   Divergent thinking, clarification, reasoning, and basic support.

Adult Health Nursing
Congestive Heart Failure

The client is a 50-year-old sales representative for a major computer company. He is married and has four children ranging in age from 13 to 18. He works long hours, rarely getting home before 8:00 PM. Two years ago, he was diagnosed with coronary artery disease after complaining of chest pain. He suffered an anterior myocardial infarction 8 months ago. Since his heart attack, the client has not successfully altered his lifestyle. Although he has reduced his work hours, he remains sedentary, continues to consume a high-fat diet, and smokes two packs of cigarettes per day.

During a visit to his physician because of fatigue and a 5-pound weight gain, he had labored respirations at 32 breaths per minute and crackles bilaterally in all lung fields. His heart rate was 120 beats per minute (bpm) with occasional irregular beats. In addition, his blood pressure was 180/110 with an S_3 noted, and he had 3 + pitting edema in his lower extremities. Upon questioning, the client stated, "I'm doing okay. I just think I need some more of those water pills you gave me a few months back."

~~~~

1. What is your initial impression of the client's physical status?

   - Review complications associated with acute myocardial infarction, such as congestive heart failure and pulmonary edema.

   - Compare the client's clinical manifestations with the classic signs and symptoms of congestive heart failure.

   - Discuss the impact of his smoking on his pulmonary and his cardiac status.

   - Draw conclusions about his complaints and physical assessment findings.

2. If the client is experiencing congestive heart failure, how will you know if he has left-sided or right-sided heart failure?

   • Compare the pathophysiological changes and clinical manifestations of right-sided heart failure to that of left-sided heart failure. List assessment findings for each.

   • Discuss additional information, such as radiology, laboratory, and electrocardiography values, that may be needed to accurately conclude which type of heart failure the client is experiencing.

3. Do the client's physical or psychosocial problems take precedence at this time?

   • Analyze the data and list the client's physical and psychosocial problems.

   • Discuss the need for addressing the client's physical problems (fluid overload, cardiac decompensation) before addressing his psychosocial problems (possible noncompliance).

   • Emphasize the need for physical stability prior to teaching.

   • Differentiate between client education and keeping the client informed of his physical status.

4. How may your biases about compliance with a treatment regimen affect the outcome of the care you deliver to that patient?

   • Identify possible biases that nurses may hold about clients who do not comply with prescribed treatment plans.

   • Speculate about how those biases may affect client care, such as treating the client in a colder manner than other patients, avoiding the patient, providing inadequate information or teaching, and labeling the patient as irresponsible or noncaring.

   • Discuss the negative connotation associated with the nursing diagnosis of noncompliance.

5. What critical thinking components did you use to answer the questions pertaining to this case?

   Divergent thinking, creativity, clarification, intellectual humility, and so on.

Adult Health Nursing
Diabetes Mellitus

The client is a 28-year-old woman who has been diabetic since the age of 8. She attends college classes in the evening while continuing her full-time day job. Recently she has been staying up late studying for final examinations. Her intense schedule has contributed to the change in her sleeping and eating patterns. Three days ago she developed influenza-like symptoms, which at first caused her little concern. Today, however, she felt worse and called her physician who instructed her to go to the emergency department.

The client's pulse and respirations were elevated, and she had a fruity odor to her breath.

The client's diagnostic findings are as follows:

Arterial blood gases: pH 7.18, $PaCO_2$ 22 mm Hg, HCO_3 10 mEq/L, PaO_2 94 mm Hg, SaO_2 98%

Chemistry profile: glucose 460 mg/dL, Na 131 mEq/L, Cl 80 mEq/L, K 5.8 mEq/L

~~~~

1. How can you explain the abnormal values from the client's arterial blood gases?

   Review the concepts of acid-base balance and imbalance, metabolic compensation, and respiratory compensation. Interpret the client's blood gases, including the type of imbalance and compensation. Discuss the relationship between the client's blood glucose level and a metabolic imbalance. Explain why she has a metabolic, as opposed to respiratory, imbalance.

2. How do you know that the client's lungs are compensating for her condition?

Discuss the concept of acid-base compensation, including the role of the lungs and kidneys in this process. Examine the client's blood gases for normal and abnormal values. Explain the collective significance of her abnormal pH, $PaCO_2$, and HCO_3.

3. What medical management interventions should you be prepared to initiate for the client?

Review the medical management of hyperglycemia, diabetic acidosis, and acid-base imbalance. Discuss the use of insulin, sodium bicarbonate, and potassium to treat the client's condition. Examine your role in each of the possible interventions.

4. Which other groups of patients have similar problems?

List types of clients who are prone to develop acid-base imbalances, such as people with malnutrition, chronic alcoholism, diarrhea, cardiac failure, and renal insufficiency. Examine how these conditions are similar. Explain why these individuals are at increased risk of developing acid-base disorders.

5. What critical thinking components did you use to address this case?

Clarification, divergent thinking, reasoning, intellectual perseverance, among others.

Adult Health Nursing
Fluid Retention of Unknown Etiology

The client is a 66-year-old woman who weighs 154 lbs and is 5 ft, 4 in tall. She lives with her retired husband. They own their own home and live with their three dogs. The client watches her 3-year-old granddaughter 2 days each week. She visited her physician today, who admitted her to the hospital for her recent weight gain of 15 lbs, shortness of breath with activity, and ankle edema. She denies recent serious illnesses, trauma, or surgery.

Assessment reveals a well-nourished female who is dyspneic, has crackles in both lower lung fields, and has 1+ pitting edema of both ankles. Her oral temperature is 99.4F, her blood pressure is 146/92, her atrial rate is 98 beats per minute (bpm) and regular, and her respiratory rate is 28 breaths per minute.

~~~~

1. Of the above data, which are most relevant to her present situation and care?

   Group data into subjective and objective problem categories. Review the case and note whether any other data are pertinent to her care. Consider her complaints, clinical manifestations, vital signs, and other assessment data.

2. What can you infer about the causes of the client's symptoms?

   Review your problem list mentioned previously. Consider the significance of the client's weight gain, her peripheral edema, and her lung sounds. Speculate about conditions that can produce these symptoms, such as chronic obstructive pulmonary disease (COPD), congestive heart failure, and renal insufficiency.

3. What further data would help you plan care for the client?

   Review the conditions that you identified previously. Identify other significant data that would support or refute your theories about the cause of her current problem. Consider obtaining an electrocardiogram, chest x-ray, arterial blood gases, serum creatinine, and blood urea nitrogen.

4. What are your priority nursing interventions for the client?

   Review the client's priority problem list. Investigate the Nursing Interventions Classification (NIC) for interventions specific to her identified problems. Consider interventions to address her dyspnea, comfort, peripheral edema, possible anxiety, and so on.

5. How would your care have differed if you had known the client's medical diagnosis?

   Review your priority interventions. Decide if your interventions could be initiated independently or require medical collaboration. Consider the care you provide to all of your clients. Consider whether you need to know a client's medical diagnosis, once his or her problems have been identified, in order to provide adequate care. Identify instances in which it is important to know the client's medical diagnosis.

6. What critical thinking components did you use to address this case?

   Divergent thinking, reasoning, creativity, basic support, and so on.

Adult Health Nursing
Hepatitis B

The client is a 28-year-old single homosexual man who recently traveled to Asia on a missionary trip. On the basis of his personal beliefs, the client signed a waiver and refused a hepatitis vaccine, even though it was highly suggested for people traveling abroad. After returning home, the client began experiencing fatigue and anorexia. When his condition failed to improve, he consulted a physician at the acquired immunodeficiency syndrome (AIDS) center where he works. Concerned that he might be positive for human immunodeficiency virus (HIV), both the physician and the client decided that a chemistry profile and HIV antibody test should be performed. The client was found to be HIV negative, but his liver-enzymes and bilirubin were elevated. Subsequently, the physician ordered serologic markers for hepatitis. Further questioning revealed that the client had been having light-colored stools and voiding dark-colored urine.

The client is currently hospitalized for treatment of hepatitis B. He denies the use of intravenous (IV) drugs or alcohol. In general, he has been well except for mild eczema and generalized pain and itching, for which he has been taking aspirin.

Upon examination, the client is somewhat slow to respond to questions and appears drowsy and lethargic. His sclera are slightly yellow, and his skin is dry with evidence of scratching; he complains of frequent itching. His abdomen is soft and nondistended. Bowel sounds are present in all four quadrants. He complains of abdominal tenderness upon palpation, abdominal discomfort, indigestion, and nausea. His urine is of adequate volume but brownish in color.

The client's diagnostic findings are as follows:

Serum markers: positive HBsAg, anti-HBcAg, HBeAg

Chemistry profile: bilirubin 5.2 mg/dL, SGPT/ALT 640 U/L, SGOT/AST 410 U/L, alkaline phosphatase 130 U/L

Coagulation: prothrombin time = 20 seconds.

~~~~

1. What is unique about the alkaline phosphatase and prothrombin time in clients with hepatitis B?

   Review the significance of abnormal values for both the alkaline phosphatase and prothrombin time. Discuss how hepatitis alters both of these laboratory findings. Compare the client's values with normal values. Compare abnormal values noted with hepatitis B with values noted in client's with other types of hepatitis, such as A or C.

2. How are the client's positive serologic markers significant to his diagnosis?

   - Compare the three serologic markers for hepatitis. Discuss the differences between the three markers that are positive in this client. Discuss the importance of each one.

   - Review the primary diagnostic indicators for each of the hepatitis groups. Compare the diagnostic indicators for hepatitis B with the client's test results.

3. What additional information would help determine the client's exposure to the hepatitis B virus?

   Review the transmission methods of hepatitis B. Speculate about possible sources of infection, such as sexual contacts, needle sticks, lacerations, and so on. Discuss methods of obtaining such information without appearing judgmental.

4. The client asks if he can continue taking aspirin or Tylenol for his generalized discomfort. Why are these medications contraindicated in this situation?

   - Review the pathophysiology of hepatitis.

   - Review the effects of Tylenol and aspirin. Examine the actions of these drugs that make them inappropriate for use by clients who have liver problems and hepatitis in particular.

   - Explore the use of alternative drugs for pain relief.

5. What is the relationship between the client's jaundice and his generalized pain and itching?

   - Review the effects of compromised hepatic function. Identify how liver dysfunction can alter skin integrity and increase generalized pain and itching.

   - Explore other conditions that can result in the same or a similar problem.

   - Examine nursing interventions that can help you reduce the client's discomfort.

6. The client is eager to recover and continue his missionary and AIDS work. What should you tell him to expect regarding his recovery?

   Examine the long-term effects of hepatitis B, including the length of recovery or potential complications. Consider the probability of the client becoming a chronic carrier and the effect it would have on his work. Identify important information that the patient should be given, including signs and symptoms of complications, use of over-the-counter and prescribed medications, recovery expectations, and the importance of close follow-up care.

7. What prejudices are possible regarding this situation? Why is it important that you understand your own prejudices when caring for any client?

   Discuss the reasons for which the client's sexual orientation place him at increased risk for discrimination. Identify other diseases or activities that place clients at risk for discrimination, such as obesity, smoking with chronic obstructive pulmonary disease (COPD), noncompliance with medical regimens, and so on. Examine the consequences to the client when you have prejudices that may affect care delivery.

8. Recall instances in which you felt you were a victim of discrimination. What types of verbal or nonverbal behavior made you feel this way?

   Discuss statements, facial expressions, or other behaviors that may indicate negativity. Encourage students to talk about how they felt during and after this experience.

9. Did the client deserve to contract hepatitis B because he refused to be immunized?

   • Argue both for and against the client's decision to refuse the hepatitis B immunization.

   • Discuss the guilt that the client may be feeling since his refusal of the vaccine.

10. What critical thinking components did you use to answer the questions pertaining to this case?

   Clarification, reasoning, intellectual sense of justice, intellectual humility, and so on.

Adult Health Nursing

Human Immunodeficiency Virus (HIV) Infection

The client is a 37-year-old divorced woman who lives with her two daughters in a rural community. She has been admitted to the hospital with complaints of fatigue, low-grade fever, night sweats, and a persistent cough. She suspects that she contracted influenza from her former boyfriend about 4 weeks ago and fears that she has developed pneumonia. She relates a history of frequent episodes of diarrhea over the past few days and sore, white patches in her mouth.

Assessment reveals a well-nourished client who appears fatigued. She has bilateral lower-lobe crackles, an oral temperature of 101.6F, a pulse of 90 beats per minute (bpm), and respirations of 32 breaths per minute, which are regular and somewhat labored. The client coughs frequently but is having difficulty expectorating anything. The nurse asks the client if she has ever had an HIV test, to which the client replies, "No, why should I?"

~~~~

1. What evidence suggests that the client could have an HIV infection or acquired immunodeficiency syndrome (AIDS)?

   • Analyze the client's complaints and physical assessment data, including her persistent cough and recent development of diarrhea. Note that she is single and has a former boyfriend. Note also that she has never had an HIV test.

   • Discuss the dangers inherent in forming conclusions without adequate evidence.

2. What further data are needed to support a diagnosis of an infection with HIV?

Review clinical manifestations, laboratory data, and risk factors associated with HIV infection. Consider the need for a social history, including information about past and current sexual activity, and laboratory data such as an Enzyme-Linked ImmunoSorbent Assay (ELISA), CD4 cell counts, HIV viral-load analysis, and so on.

3. How can you respond appropriately to the client's comment about HIV testing?

Review the legal and ethical implications of suggesting that someone has HIV. Discuss the need for the client to provide permission before her physician can order an HIV test. Consider how you would feel if you were in the client's position. Devise alternative ways of obtaining information from the client without suggesting that she has HIV.

4. On the basis of the client's clinical manifestations, why should you suspect that the client has AIDS?

Review the criteria given by the Centers for Disease Control for the diagnosis and classification of AIDS. Identify the clinical manifestations that support a diagnosis of AIDS in this case, as opposed to HIV infection. Consider the possible presence of three opportunistic infections, such as pneumocystis pneumonia, cryptosporidiosis, and oral candidiasis.

5. What critical thinking components did you use to address this case?

Creativity, clarification, intellectual empathy, among others.

Adult Health Nursing
Hyperthyroidism

The client is a 40-year-old single mother of two children. She works as a high-school counselor and is a member of the city council. The client was diagnosed with hyperthyroidism (Grave's disease) and is being admitted to the hospital for I^{131} treatment. She is extremely anxious about the procedure as well as the results it will produce.

The client sees her family physician annually for a physical examination and has been generally well for the past several years. About 8 months ago, however, she noted a general feeling of nervousness, irritability, and pounding heartbeat. Thinking these symptoms were related to stress, she did not become concerned. Over the following weeks, the client noticed that she seemed to be less tolerant of the summer heat and was eating more than usual while continuing to lose weight. Realizing she was due for a general physical examination, she scheduled an office visit with her family physician. She has no known allergies to foods or medications.

Upon examination, the client is alert, oriented, and cooperative but obviously restless. She has mild protrusion of the eyes (exophthalmos), complains of pho-tophobia, and has a palpable smooth symmetrical goiter. Her oral temperature is 99.8F, her pulse is regular at 120 beats per minute (bpm), and her respiratory rate is also regular at 18 breaths per minute. She complains of slight shortness of breath with exertion. Her blood pressure is 180/92. She has no jugular vein distention, peripheral edema, or abnormal lung sounds. Her skin is warm and flushed, and her nails are thin and friable. The client is 5 ft, 4 in tall and weighs 105 lbs.

The client's diagnostic findings are as follows:

Thyroid studies: elevated T_3, T_4, TSH, and BMR

~~~~~

1. What is the connection between the client's exophthalmos, rapid pulse, and weight loss and her disease process?

   Review the function of the thyroid gland and changes that occur with the loss of its normal function. Address the impact of hyperthyroidism on metabolic rate and the loss of homeostatic mechanisms. Discuss clinical manifestations that occur with reversible and nonreversible treatments.

2. Why should the client undergo a cardiac assessment?

   Discuss the impact of a hyperactive thyroid on body organs, particularly the heart. Identify data that support the need for a cardiac assessment, such as the client's increased blood pressure and heart rate. Speculate about possible consequences of not performing a cardiac assessment.

3. What are the client's priority nursing diagnoses while she is hospitalized and undergoing treatment?

   Review the data in this case. Consider the client's anxiety about the radioactive iodine treatments, her concerns about the outcome of the procedure, possible side effects of the radioactive iodine treatments, and the impact of radiation precautions on her anxiety. Discuss nursing diagnoses that address her concerns as well as her physical needs.

4. What can you do to alleviate the client's anxiety while maintaining the precautions necessary for her treatment?

   Discuss the use of the Nursing Interventions Classification (NIC) for addressing the client's priority nursing diagnoses. Consider radiation therapy management, anxiety reduction, and client teaching about the disease process and prescribed medications. Select appropriate activities for the client's situation. Investigate hospital policies regarding the use of radioactive iodine and recommended precautions for clients and health care providers.

5. How are chemical obliteration of the thyroid gland and hypothyroidism similar?

   Review the disease process of hypothyroidism and the effect of decreased thyroid hormone on all body systems. Compare the changes associated with the disease to those changes that are likely to occur from chemical obliteration.

6. What criteria can be used to determine if the client will require special eye care?

   Review the pathophysiology of exophthalmos and its effect on the client's comfort and vision. Consider clinical manifestations that require long-term treatment because they are permanent versus those that may require short-term treatment because they will resolve when the client's thyroid levels return to normal.

7. How can you generalize the client's care to clients with other hormonal disturbances, such as hypothyroidism, adrenal insufficiency, Cushing's syndrome, or diabetes mellitus?

   Discuss the client's primary nursing diagnoses and how they might apply to other patients. Consider her fear of her treatment outcome, anxiety over the treatment, potential permanency of a physical defect (exophthalmos), ability to adjust to a chronic illness and a lifetime of medication, and so on.

8. What critical thinking components did you use to answer the questions pertaining to this case?

   Intellectual empathy, reasoning, clarification, divergent thinking, and so on.

Adult Health Nursing
Living with a Cardiac Pacemaker

The client is a 56-year-old man who is being discharged from the hospital following the insertion of a demand pacemaker. This device is necessary to treat his symptomatic bradycardia and second-degree heart block. The client is a truck driver and is concerned about how the pacemaker will affect his ability to continue working. He enjoys weight lifting, hunting, and working on his antique automobiles. He and his wife enjoy traveling and are planning a trip to Asia in several months. Both voice concern that they will have to cancel their trip and make major lifestyle changes to accomodate the client's condition, including disposing of their microwave oven and avoiding gardening, swimming, and other physical activities.

~~~~

1. What is the relationship between bradycardia, second-degree heart block, and the need for a pacemaker?

   - Review the pathophysiology of second-degree heart block and associated bradycardia. Note the possible consequences of severe bradycardia such as dizziness, loss of consciousness, or death. Review the function of a pacemaker.

   - Discuss the concept of "demand" pacing versus "fixed-rate pacing." Explain how the client's pacemaker will allow his heart to maintain adequate circulation.

2. Are the client's fears about lifestyle changes realistic?

Review precautions that are necessary following the insertion of a permanent pacemaker. Identify contraindicated and acceptable activities. Determine the client's interests and activities that may have to change, such as hunting, use of equipment that may not be grounded, and weight lifting. Explore the reasons why such activities are contraindicated. Decide whether the client's fears are realistic.

3. What are the priority teaching needs for this couple?

Identify the teaching needs for this couple regarding follow-up care, use of electrical equipment, exercise, and so on. Consider informing the client that travel is not prohibited, contemporary microwave ovens are not hazardous to pacemakers, wearing identification is recommended, and keeping scheduled follow-up appointments is important.

4. How would you feel if you were told that you would have to alter your present lifestyle?

Identify lifestyle changes that would be easy and difficult to make. Identify factors that make lifestyle changes easy or difficult. Discuss the degree to which client education fosters compliance with recommended lifestyle changes.

5. What critical thinking components did you use to address this case?

Reasoning, reflection, basic support, intellectual empathy, among others.

Adult Health Nursing
Multiple Sclerosis

The client went to her physician's office approximately 3 years ago with complaints of weakness, fatigue, and occasional loss of muscle ability. She complained that she would frequently drop things for no reason. Additionally, she had experienced nystagmus and transient diplopia. Her physician ordered extensive diagnostic studies that eventually led to the diagnosis of multiple sclerosis. She was placed on 40 mg of prednisone daily and the muscle relaxant baclofen. Her condition stabilized, and she was released with minimal dysfunction.

Approximately 1 month ago, the client's sister died in an automobile accident. While they did not live near one another, the client's sister had been a significant source of support. Since her sister's death, the client has noticed a significant increase in her fatigue and muscle weakness. Her gait has become unsteady, and she has fallen on several occasions. It has become increasingly difficult for her to perform her job responsibilities. Last week her employer requested that she take a leave of absence and apply for permanent disability.

Yesterday the client was admitted to the hospital with spastic weakness of her extremities, intention tremors, dysphagia, and urinary incontinence. She is withdrawn and cries frequently. Her physical assessment reveals a blood pressure of 110/76, a heart rate of 82 beats per minute (bpm), a respiratory rate of 24 breaths per minute, an oral temperature of 98.6F, weight of 118 lbs, and height of 5 ft, 6 in. Her skin is warm and dry. She is lethargic and unable to lift her glass without spilling its contents. She complains of severe muscle spasms in both lower legs, and she is unaware that she is experiencing urinary incontinence. Her physician feels that she has chronic relapsing-remitting multiple sclerosis.

~~~~

1. What conclusions can you draw about the client's current health status?

   Cluster data into related categories. Draw conclusions about each data cluster. Consider her recent stressful event, exacerbation of clinical manifestations, physical findings, and so on.

2. What further data do you need to support your conclusions?

   Review your data clusters. Decide what further data are needed to support the conclusions you drew previously about each category. Consider laboratory data, medical history, other assessment findings, and so on.

3. Why is multiple sclerosis considered an autoimmune disease?

   Review the concept of autoimmunity. Review the pathophysiology of multiple sclerosis. Discuss the immune reaction that occurs with multiple sclerosis. Summarize the characteristics that classify multiple sclerosis as an autoimmune disease.

4. Why are some forms of multiple sclerosis characterized by periods of remission and exacerbation?

   Review the pathophysiology of multiple sclerosis, noting the characteristic pattern of inflammation and destruction that takes place along the myelin sheaths of nerve cells. Discuss the direct relationship between inflammation along the myelin sheath and symptom production. Explain how reducing inflammation can decrease symptoms.

5. How do the various forms of multiple sclerosis differ?

   Review the various classifications of multiple sclerosis. Compare each type on the basis of its onset, rapidity of progression, length of remissions, prognosis, and so on. List clinical manifestations that occur with each form of multiple sclerosis. Identify similarities and differences.

6. What impact did the death of the client's sister have on her current illness?

   Explain the physical and psychosocial effects of stress on clients suffering from autoimmune diseases. Identify the relationship between increased stress and exacerbation of multiple sclerosis.

7. How is the drug prednisone beneficial to patients like this client?

   Research the effects of prednisone on the inflammatory process. Discuss the need to reduce inflammation along the myelin sheath in order to reduce clinical manifestations. Discuss the concept of immunosuppression. Explain why immunosuppression is beneficial to clients with autoimmune diseases.

8. How would you prioritize nursing care for the client?

   Cluster physical and psychological data into related categories. Identify the most appropriate nursing diagnoses for your data clusters. Considering the client's present state, use a framework to prioritize the nursing diagnoses and interventions for each diagnosis, such as the life-preservation framework.

9. How can you generalize the care of this client to other clients with autoimmune diseases?

   Identify common characteristics of classic autoimmune diseases, such as lupus erythematosus, rheumatoid arthritis, systemic sclerosis, and so on. Consider clinical manifestations, exacerbating factors, nursing care, and medical management of these diseases.

10. What are your biases concerning the client's employer asking her to quit her job and apply for disability benefits?

    Consider your negative and positive biases. Consider how you might feel if you were the client. Imagine how you might feel if you were her employer. List your biases.

11. What attitude and cognitive critical thinking skills did you use to address this case?

Basic support, divergent thinking, reasoning, intellectual humility, among others.

Adult Health Nursing
Renal Calculi

The client is a 45-year-old man who, while sitting at his desk at work, experiences sudden, severe back pain on his left side. He walks about the room for awhile but receives no relief from the pain. After about 30 minutes, he asks his coworker to take him to the emergency department because he can no longer tolerate the pain. Upon arrival, the client's pain is excruciating; he is unable to lie still on the emergency department cart. The client is cold, clammy, diaphoretic, and pale. His blood pressure is 100/70, his pulse is 94 beats per minute (bpm), his respirations are 28 breaths per minute, and his oral temperature is 98.8F. The client denies ever having this type of pain in the past or a history of kidney stones. The physician, suspecting renal calculi, orders an intravenous (IV) infusion of lactated Ringer's solution, 10 mg of IV morphine sulfate, and an IV pyelogram.

~~~~

1. What are the advantages of thinking through the client's problem before making a decision about the cause of his pain?

   Discuss the benefit of collecting adequate data prior to making decisions. Discuss the consequences to the client if treatment is initiated for a problem that he does not have or if treatment is not initiated because of inadequate data collection. Consider consequences such as increased pain, potential physical complications, increased costs, and so on.

2. What is the relationship between the client's present physical status (decreased blood pressure, cold, clammy skin, and so on.) and his pain?

Compare and contrast acute with chronic pain. Note the effect of severe, acute pain on normal physiology. Identify aspects of the stress response that result in symptoms commonly associated with shock. Compare your findings with the client's conditions. Consider your own past experiences with pain, particularly those that made you feel physically ill.

3. Why should you administer IV fluids to the client?

Examine common treatments for renal calculi. Consider the need to flush calculi from the kidney into the ureter and the need to dilate the ureter so that calculi can pass with greater ease. Discuss the need to eliminate the kidney stone in order to reduce pain.

4. How can the client be suffering from renal calculi if he has no previous history of kidney stones?

Review the pathophysiology and contributing factors to the development of renal calculi. Consider the size of calculi and the need for the calculi to enter the ureter in order to produce symptoms. Consider that many people do not know they are at risk for, or actually have, some diseases until problems occur, such as renal calculi, hypertension, cardiac disease, and so on.

5. What critical thinking components did you use to address this case?

Clarification, reflection, basic support, faith in reason, and so on.

Adult Health Nursing
Respiratory Compromise Following Hip Surgery

The client is a 68-year-old woman who relates a history of congestive heart failure and osteoarthritis. Two days ago she underwent a right total hip replacement. Since her surgery, she has had difficulty coughing up secretions. A few minutes ago the client called the nurse to her room complaining of shortness of breath and a "tight" feeling in her chest. She is pale and diaphoretic, has an irregular apical rate of 125 beats per minute (bpm), a labored respiratory rate of 28 breaths per minute, and a blood pressure of 142/90. She is obviously anxious and states, "Please help me. I think I'm dying."

~~~~

1. What is your first impression of the client's physical status?

   Review both the client's objective and subjective data. Identify priority problems. Consider possibilities such as anxiety, fear, airway compromise due to thick secretions, pulmonary embolism, atelectasis, and pneumothorax.

2. What further data are necessary to better assess the client's situation?

   Review objective and subjective data and identify information that is missing or that needs to be ordered by the physician. Consider lung sounds; appearance of lung secretions; and the need for obtaining arterial blood gases, a chest x-ray, and hemoglobin and hematocrit levels.

3. What evidence suggests that oxygen delivery to the tissues has been compromised?

   Analyze the client's clinical manifestations and identify those that are significant for compromised oxygenation. Consider her vital signs, increased heart rate and respirations, and quality of respirations. Discuss the benefits and possible detriments of tachycardia and tachypnea.

4. How does hip replacement surgery place the patient at increased risk for compromised oxygenation?

   Discuss the possible consequences of bone manipulation, such as blood clot formation and fatty embolism. Discuss the need for maximizing oxygenation to prevent stasis of secretions and atelectasis.

5. How can the nurse best respond to the client's feeling that she is dying?

   Consider how you might feel if you were in the client's situation. Identify nursing activities that would help you feel secure versus those that would reinforce your feelings of anxiety. Consider staying with the client, using touch, and talking in a soothing reassuring voice. Discuss the possible impact of statements such as, "Don't worry, you're going to be okay" or "calm down, I'm going for help."

6. What critical thinking components did you use to address this case?

   Divergent thinking, reasoning, creativity, intellectual empathy, and so on.

Adult Health Nursing
Spinal Cord Injury

The client is an 18-year-old man who suffered a spinal cord injury at the level of C-5 during a boating accident. He is currently in a rehabilitation setting with assisted ventilation and quadriplegia. He has a reflex neurogenic bladder that fills and empties automatically. The nursing staff is teaching the client's 17-year-old wife techniques to facilitate bladder emptying and intermittent catheterization. The client is also on a bowel retraining program that includes stool softeners to prevent fecal impaction. At times the client's wife seems overwhelmed with her husband's problems, but she is supportive and asks numerous questions.

One afternoon following lunch, the client begins to complain of a throbbing headache. The nurse notes that his forehead is wet with perspiration and his face is flushed. His blood pressure is 250/160, his pulse is 58 beats per minute (bpm) and regular, his respirations are 24 breaths per minute, his oral temperature is 99.8F, and his extremities are cool and pale. His wife is alarmed and wants you to do something immediately.

~~~~

1. What inferences can you make about the client's physical condition and current problem?

   Review complications associated with spinal cord injury. Compare clinical manifestations of suspected complications with the client's clinical manifestations. Consider possible problems, especially autonomic dysreflexia.

2. What are the causes or contributing factors to the client's current problem?

Discuss the pathophysiology of autonomic dysreflexia and its relationship to spinal cord injury. List factors that contribute to its development. Identify the client's risk factors for the development of autonomic dysreflexia. Consider distended urinary bladder, fecal impaction, bladder infection, suppository insertion, tight clothing, and so on.

3. What priority nursing interventions should you implement for the client?

Review nursing care for the client experiencing autonomic dysreflexia. Consider interventions such as elevating the head of his bed, removing the offending stimulus such as the urinary catheter, checking his urinary bladder for distention and/or fullness, and checking for rectal impaction.

4. If you were the client's wife, how could the nurse best help you?

Evaluate your ability to deal with the client and his wife's situation as a 17-year-old. Examine the developmental stage of a 17-year-old and predict the success of her ability to assume responsibility for her husband. Consider interventions that are both supportive and beneficial, such as teaching, allowing the client's wife to participate in his care, discussing alternatives for care, offering information about referrals, and so on.

5. What critical thinking components did you use to address this case?

Basic support, clarification, reflection, intellectual empathy, and so on.

Adult Health Nursing
Systemic Lupus Erythematosus

For approximately 5 years the client has been under a physician's care for discoid and systemic lupus erythematosus. Initially her physician prescribed steroid creams for her facial rash and oral nonsteroidal anti-inflammatory drugs (NSAIDs) for joint pain. Her symptoms have been well controlled until recently.

Three days ago, the client was admitted to the hospital with the primary complaint of acute joint pain. Her physical assessment revealed a blood pressure of 180/104, a heart rate of 100 beats per minute (bpm), a respiratory rate of 28 breaths per minute, an oral temperature of 100.6F. She weighed 140 lbs, and was 5 ft, 4 in tall. The client's skin was pink, dry, and warm. Her knee and wrist joints, in particular, were warm, swollen, and tender. She was oriented to person, place, and time and in obvious acute pain; she was quiet and somewhat withdrawn. Her lung sounds were clear, bowel sounds were present in four quadrants, and her abdomen was nondistended. In addition, her pedal pulses were strong bilaterally.

The client has been placed on bed rest with bathroom privileges, ice packs to wrists and knees, 500 mg of naproxen every 12 hours, 20 mg of prednisone three times a day, and diet as tolerated. A routine urinalysis revealed protein in her urine.

~~~~

1. What conclusions can you draw about the client's current health status?

   Cluster data into related categories. Analyze your data clusters for patterns. Consider the client's clinical manifestations, her primary concerns, the medications she is taking, her laboratory data, and so on.

2. What other data would be helpful when planning care for the client?

Review your data clusters. Identify data that are missing. Consider family history, exacerbating factors, laboratory data such as blood urea nitrogen and serum creatinine, autoantibody studies, serum complement, and so on. Explain why this information is relevant to the client's care.

3. How does discoid lupus erythematosus differ from systemic lupus erythematosus?

Investigate both discoid and systemic lupus erythematosus. Note the similarities and differences between the two conditions. Consider the degree of connective-tissue involvement, the extent of disease, complications, management, and so on.

4. What are the priority nursing interventions for this client?

Using your data clusters from question 1, identify nursing diagnoses that address each problem. Using the life-preservation framework or similar tool, prioritize the client's nursing diagnoses. Decide which interventions are most appropriate for each nursing diagnosis you selected.

5. How will ice affect the client's pain status?

Research the use of ice for inflammation. Discuss the components of the inflammatory response that are beneficially suppressed by the use of ice, such as increased blood flow.

6. Why is lupus erythematosus considered a classic example of an autoimmune disease?

Review the concept of autoimmunity. Review the pathophysiology and defining characteristics of systemic lupus erythematosus. Discuss the detrimental effects of immune destruction of the body's own cells occurring with systemic lupus erythematosus.

7. How will you know if the client's medication therapy is effective?

   Research the desired effects of steroids and NSAIDs on inflammation. Identify clinical manifestations that will be reduced or resolved as a result of medication therapy. Explain how immunosuppression may reduce or control autoimmune destruction.

8. What concerns should you have about administering prednisone with NSAIDs?

   • Review the actions and interactions of the drug prednisone and NSAIDs. Explain why such drug interactions are a concern to the nurse and client.

   • Identify parameters (assessment findings) indicative of drug interactions.

9. What is the significance of the client's urinalysis?

   Review the pathophysiology of systemic lupus erythematosus. Discuss the common complications of this disease, such as glomerular disease, on the basis of your research of its pathophysiology. Explain how immune complex formation can alter glomerular filtration.

10. What critical thinking attitude and cognitive skills did you use to address this case?

   Divergent thinking, clarification, basic support, and intellectual perseverance.

Community and Home Care Nursing

Community and Home Care Nursing
Acquired Immunodeficiency Syndrome (AIDS)

The client is a 42-year-old with symptomatic human immunodeficiency virus (HIV) disease (AIDS), who lives with his partner and caregiver. The client is a writer who works from home and has a large network of supportive family members and friends. The home health nurse visits twice weekly to assess the client's physical status and help with his numerous medications. In addition to antiretroviral drugs, the client takes herbal supplements and smokes marijuana to stimulate his appetite. His CD4 T cell count recently dropped from 500 to $420/mm^3$.

During a routine visit, the nurse notices a dry cough and hears crackles in both lung bases. The client is wrapped in a blanket and complains of being cold even though the room temperature is normal. He admits to mild dyspnea for the past 2 days but states, "I didn't tell anyone because I don't want to go back into the hospital." His blood pressure is 150/90, his heart rate is 106 beats per minute (bpm) and regular, his respiratory rate is 28 breaths per minute and regular, and his oral temperature is 101.8F.

~~~~

1. What can you infer from the client's assessment findings?

   - Cluster relevant data into categories.

   - Identify problems suggested by the data clusters. Consider the possibility of an opportunistic infection, resistance to his medications, and so on.

   - Review your inferences. Decide if they are justified by the data or if you need more information.

2. What is the significance of the client's CD4 T cell count?

   • Review the relationship between CD4 T cell counts and HIV infection.

   • Discuss complications that can occur when T cells are extensively reduced.

   • Relate the client's T cell count to his present symptoms.

3. What other information would be helpful when planning care for the client?

   • Review your data clusters.

   • Decide which data are missing to confirm your suspicions about the cause of the client's current symptoms and help you plan his care. Consider performing further assessments to determine the client's mental status, cardiac status, gastrointestinal (GI) status, and so on, obtaining more information about his medical history; and researching his current medications other than the antiretroviral medications.

4. What nursing interventions will be most useful to the client?

   • Review home care of a client with an opportunistic infection.

   • Decide which nursing activities would be most beneficial in reducing the client's discomfort and enhancing his breathing ability. Consider the need to obtain further medical attention for the client and how to best approach the client in this regard.

5. Why do you think the client is reluctant to report his infection to his primary care provider?

   Discuss both the physical and psychosocial aspects of AIDS and the need for frequent home care and hospitalization. Consider the client's possible concerns such as ineffectiveness of medication, progression of the disease, increased debility; and fear of death.

6. What critical thinking attitudes and cognitive skills did you use to address this case?

   Divergent thinking, reasoning, intellectual perseverance, intellectual humility, and so on.

Community and Home Care Nursing
Alzheimer's Disease

The client is a 67-year-old woman who resides with her husband at home. The client and her husband have been married for 47 years and have raised two sons who live in distant states. They have no family in the immediate area who can help them. The couple is on a fixed income and have little savings. The client is a retired school teacher, and her husband recently retired from the police force. They were active in their local church until the client began exhibiting disturbing behaviors that made it difficult for her husband to take her to church functions.

The client was recently diagnosed with Alzheimer's disease. She also has a history of a cerebrovascular accident that left her with right-sided weakness. She was healthy until about 4 years ago when her husband began to notice that she was becoming forgetful. For a while the client was able to mask her forgetfulness by using calendars and Post-it notes, but it soon became apparent that her memory loss was impacting her ability to function on a day-to-day basis.

The client's diagnosis has been difficult for her husband. He is supportive of his wife and becomes tearful when he thinks about how life used to be. Last week his wife did not recognize him, which was particularly traumatic for him. He is having difficulty caring for the client because she recently became incontinent of urine and verbally aggressive, sometimes striking at him. He confesses that sometimes he feels like striking back.

The client no longer takes his wife anywhere because he fears she will embarrass him. He is unable to leave her alone in the house because he is afraid that she will wander outside and become lost. She wakes him throughout the night, which adds to his fatigue. He readily admits his frustration with the situation.

The home health nurse finds that the client is able to state her name but is unable to recall her address or phone number. The client is evasive and unable to answer most questions. She cannot sit still for the physical assessment and paces the room. She repeatedly asks the nurse why he is there. The nurse notices several bruises on the client's arms and legs. When questioned, the client's husband states that she is careless and frequently stumbles when she walks. He does not seem concerned. The client's blood pressure is 90/60, her oral temperature is 98.4F, her heart rate is 88 beats per minute (bpm), and her respirations are 24 breaths per minute.

Her medications include one 2.5-mg tablet of Coumadin daily, one tablet of multivitamin daily, and one 40-mg tablet of propranolol daily.

~~~~

1. What conclusions can you draw about the client's health status?

   - Review the data, noting her assessment findings, her current and past medical history, and the additional information provided from her husband.

   - List possible conclusions about the client's bruising, such as spouse abuse, medication-related causes, and the validity of the husband's explanations. Decide if your conclusions are based on the facts of the case or assumptions triggered by your feelings.

2. What further data do you need to support your conclusions?

   - Review the data and your conclusions.

   - For those conclusions not supported by data, identify additional information that would support or refute your conclusions. Consider the client's medications, past CVA, and so forth.

3. What factors place the client at increased risk for bruising?

   - Review data that support risk for falls, such as her right-sided weakness and her medication therapy.

   - Research the mechanisms of action and possible side effects of Coumadin and propranolol.

   - Discuss the relationship between Coumadin and bruising.

4. Of what significance is the client's low blood pressure?

   - Review the client's data, especially her medications.

   - Identify medications that affect blood pressure.

   - Decide if she could be experiencing postural hypotension.

   - Discuss the effect of propranolol.

   - Explore the relationship between hypotension and risk for falls.

5. Which of the client's priority needs can be addressed by the home health nurse?

   - Cluster data into related categories and identify the client's needs.

   - Using a theoretical framework such as life preservation, prioritize the client's needs.

   - Decide which of the needs can be addressed immediately by the home health nurse and which ones will require collaboration with other health-team professionals.

6. From your knowledge of available community resources, which services may help the client's husband care for his wife at home?

   - Investigate the availability of community services in your area. Decide which of the services may provide physical or emotional relief for the client's husband.

   - Discuss the North American Nursing Diagnosis Association (NANDA) diagnosis of care-giver strain and how it applies in this case.

7. What attitude and cognitive critical thinking skills did you use to address this case?

   Basic support, divergent thinking, and so on.

Community and Home Care Nursing
Central Line Care

The client is a 32-year-old woman with insulin-dependent diabetes mellitus and a history of alcohol and intravenous (IV) drug abuse. She is familiar with her disease process but does not take care of herself. For example, she was hospitalized for several weeks with an infected plantar ulcer and eventually had a left transmetatarsal amputation. Because of recurring osteomyelitis, she was transferred to an extended care facility for 6 weeks of IV antibiotics administered through a central line.

On the final day of her IV therapy, the client left the extended care facility without waiting to have her central line removed. Her abrupt departure caused a great deal of concern because of her history of IV drug use. The physician contacted the home health nurse because of her long-standing relationship with the client. By talking to family and friends, the nurse found the client at a motel where she was living with a friend.

~~~~

1. What is your first impression of the client and her situation?

   Consider biases that influence your first impression, such as her disregard for her own health, her contribution to her own illness, her addiction that interferes with her ability to accept health care, and general biases about people with socially unacceptable habits.

2. What additional information do you need about the client before drawing conclusions about her situation?

Consider information regarding financial resources, social or family support systems, the client's current use of drugs, availability of drug rehabilitation, the client's willingness to seek such services, status of her surgical wound, status of her subclavian line and insertion site, evidence of infection, and so on.

3. Should the client's physical or psychosocial needs take priority?

- Cluster data into physical and psychosocial categories.

- Identify problems within each category.

- Speculate about the consequences of not addressing each identified problem.

- Prioritize the client's problems.

4. What critical thinking attitude and cognitive skills did you use to answer the questions in this case?

Divergent thinking, reasoning, intellectual humility, faith in reason, among others.

Community and Home Care Nursing
Choosing to Die

The client is a 94-year-old American Indian who lives with his daughter and her family in the inner city. The client follows his traditional religious practices. He has been in relatively good health until this week when he announced to his family that he is going to die. Quite concerned, his daughter contacted the clinic, and the physician there requested a visit from a home health care nurse.

The nurse finds the client lying on his bed. He is alert and cooperative. Physical assessment reveals no abnormal findings; his blood pressure is 138/90, his respiratory rate is 16 breaths per minute and regular, his pulse is 70 beats per minute (bpm) and regular, and his oral temperature is 97.8F. The client calmly states, "I've had a long life, and it is time to die." He further states that he does not want any help or treatment. He has refused food for several days but does take occasional sips of water.

The nurse discusses the situation at length with the client's family, including the fact that he is oriented and able to make decisions for himself. The family members do not want to interfere with the client's wishes and decide to allow him to continue without food. They also agree to invite other family members and friends over to spend time with the client before he dies. Two days later, the daughter calls to thank the nurse and inform him that the client died in his sleep.

~~~~

1. How do you feel about this situation?

   - Examine your feelings about quality of life and death.

   - Explore the differences between cultures and their views about death.

   - Identify your own biases about interfering with the client's choice to die.

   - Consider the sorrow, guilt, or other emotions that you may feel in this situation.

2. What are some of the cultural issues depicted in this situation?

   • Consider the client's state of health, his belief that it was time to die, and so on.

   • Discuss the goal of health care.

   • Discuss the conflict that occurs between nurses and clients when they have cultural differences.

3. Do you think the nurse did the right thing in this instance?

   • Consider potential biases in this case, such as those against the family for not intervening to save the client or the bias that people who opt to die are mentally incompetent, and so on.

   • Consider whether a person should have the right to die as he or she chooses.

4. How would you present the opposite perspective?

   • Depending on how question 3 was answered, present the other side of the argument.

   • Identify facts, beliefs, or opinions that influence your argument in either direction.

5. Compare the responsibilities of the home health nurse to those of the acute care nurse when dealing with cultural differences?

   • Review concepts of client advocacy and client rights.

   • Explore how these concepts apply to both the hospital and home settings.

   • Identify the importance of nurses becoming familiar with other cultures, in order to avoid placing the nurse's cultural values above the client's values.

6. What critical thinking attitudes and cognitive skills did you use to address this case?

   Intellectual courage, sense of justice, divergent thinking, clarification, and so on.

Community and Home Care Nursing
Chronic Obstructive Pulmonary Disease (COPD)

The client is an 82-year-old retired widower who lives by himself in a small home. His son lives nearby and provides emotional and limited financial support. The client is homebound due to obesity and exertional dyspnea. He smoked two packs of cigarettes for more than 20 years, although he has not smoked for the past 3 years. He has COPD and a history of heart disease. His current medications include 20 mg of lovastatin every day for hyperlipidemia, 2 puffs of albuterol from an inhaler 4 times a day, and 325 mg of ASA every day.

Currently, the client's physician is treating him for an upper respiratory infection, which involves a sore throat, fever, and cough producing thick, yellow sputum. The client has been placed on 500 mg of erythromycin 4 times a day for 10 days. Because the client has difficulty getting to the office, the physician requested a home health nurse to assess the client's respiratory status on the third day after initiating treatment.

The examination reveals much improvement in the client's respiratory condition. However, he complains of muscle aches, weakness, and difficulty getting out of bed. His blood pressure is 134/88, his pulse is 84 beats per minute (bpm) and regular, his respirations are 18 per minute with decreased breath sounds, and his oral temperature is 98.4 F.

~~~~~

1. What is your first impression of the client's situation?

   Identify possible physiological, psychological, and sociological problems. Consider your first impressions, such as the client may be experiencing complications related to his respiratory infection, may be suffering from medication interaction, may be incompetent to care for himself independently, and so forth.

2. What conclusions can you draw on the basis of the client's data?

- Analyze subjective and objective data and create a list identifying the client's most significant problems.

- From this list, draw conclusions on the basis of the data as opposed to your assumptions or feelings.

3. What are the possible causes of the client's clinical manifestations in view of his improved respiratory status?

- Investigate the effects, side effects, toxicity, and drug interactions produced by each of the client's prescribed medications.

- Explore the relationship between his clinical manifestations and complications produced by COPD. Consider possibilities such as post flu syndrome, medication toxicity, drug interactions, and so on.

4. How can the nurse best intervene to assist the client?

- Consider the need for further physical assessment before planning any actions. Assess the client's dietary intake; his medication regimen, including over-the-counter preparations; and the relationship of these factors to his current complaints.

- Research the interaction between the medications lovastatin and erythromycin.

- Identify actual or potential nursing diagnoses for this client. Plan appropriate actions to address each actual or potential nursing diagnosis. Discuss the use of the Nursing Interventions Classification (NIC) to address each identified nursing diagnosis.

5. What impact does the client's obesity have on his current condition?

Investigate the impact of obesity on COPD and respiratory compromise such as infection. Consider the client's inability to expand lungs, decreased mobility on lung compromise, the higher incidence of cardiac compromise, and so on.

6. How do the responsibilities of the home health nurse differ from the acute care nurse?

   Compare and contrast home health nurses and acute care nurses regarding assessments; the availability of diagnostic tests and equipment, such as pulse oximetry, limited time with clients, and so on.

7. What exercises can you suggest to the client that will not compromise his respiratory or cardiac status?

   Review low-impact or low metabolic equivalent exercises that can result in increased endurance without producing dyspnea, such as deep-breathing and range-of-motion exercises, ankle circles, walking aided by another person or a walker, and so on.

8. What is the relationship between the client's respiratory status and his cardiac disease?

   Review the physiology of the cardiac and respiratory systems and how compromise of one system can compromise the other. Consider the impact of chronically decreased oxygenation on the heart, energy level, muscle tone, and so on.

9. What biases could affect the client's care?

   - Reflect on your feelings about this case. Identify your biases.

   - Discuss characteristics of the client's case that may be viewed as socially acceptable, such as smoking or obesity.

   - Examine how such biases may impact your care, for example, the belief that the client is irresponsible or caused his own disease; he is too difficult to care for because of his size; he does not care about himself; he is sloppy because he is obese, and so on.

10. What critical thinking attitudes and skills did you use to address this case?

    Intellectual humility, intellectual empathy, reflection, clarification, and so on.

Community and Home Care Nursing
Colostomy

The client is a 59-year-old man who lives with his partner in a modest suburban home. The client has no chronic health problems other than a long history of diverticulitis and irritable bowel syndrome, which has progressively worsened over the past 2 years. Ten days ago he developed a complete bowel obstruction and was hospitalized for an emergency bowel resection. Placement of a permanent sigmoid colostomy was necessary.

The client tolerated surgery well, and his postoperative recovery was free of complications. However, he refused to learn about ostomy care and would not even look at the site. Fortunately, his partner was receptive to learning and quickly adapted to caring for the client's ostomy. He was discharged after 4 days with plans for follow-up visits from a home health nurse.

Upon the first visit to the client's home, the nurse was greeted by his partner, a plump, cheerful woman. The client was sitting in the living room watching television in his bathrobe. As the nurse asked questions about his health history and surgery, the client let his partner do most of the talking. When asked if he had been changing the ostomy appliance, the client shook his head and looked away. His partner added, "He still won't look at it, and he can't put his clothes on because it keeps leaking. I don't see how he will ever be able to go to work again." She leans toward the nurse and whispers, "I can't even leave the house because he wouldn't know what to do if the bag fell off." The client works as an accountant and needs to return to his job in time for tax season, which is a month away.

While assessing the client, the nurse asks him about his job, accounting, and income taxes. When she mentions returning to work, the client admits that he is worried about "accidents" and odors from the colostomy. "Maybe I should just take an early retirement," he adds. The nurse teaches him about bowel control and asks him if he would like to meet someone else with an ostomy. He reluctantly agrees. Then the nurse places several booklets about colostomy next to the client's chair and asks him to read them before the next visit.

The physical examination reveals normal vital signs and a healing incision. The client has active bowel sounds, shows no abdominal distention, and reports soft brown stools through the ostomy several times a day. There is some redness and several blisters on the skin surrounding the ostomy.

~ ~ ~ ~

1. What can you infer about the client's acceptance of his colostomy?

   Analyze the data to determine patterns indicative of the client's acceptance or rejection of his colostomy. Consider his silence, aversion to inspecting his colostomy, refusal to assume responsibility for it, and so on.

2. How would you evaluate the appearance of the client's colostomy?

   Compare the description of the client's colostomy with a textbook description or photograph of a healing or noncomplicated colostomy. Discuss the significance of the reddened, blistered skin around his colostomy. Consider the possibility of an ill-fitting collection system that permits leakage of stool onto the skin.

3. Considering the client's aversion to his colostomy, what kind of knowledge deficits do you suspect the client has about his colostomy?

   Identify teaching that is necessary for any person with a new colostomy, including techniques on changing the bag, controlling odor, cleaning the colostomy appliance, caring for the skin around the colostomy, and selecting the most appropriate collection system.

4. What nutritional advice is most appropriate for the client?

- Review basic principles of nutrition and consider ways of planning a balanced diet.

- Relate the type of the client's colostomy to nutrition and bowel-control techniques. Consider advice regarding foods that are most likely to cause constipation, diarrhea, odor, or flatus.

- Advise the client about introducing new foods one at a time to determine tolerance.

5. How can you effectively address the client's concern about the leakage and odor produced by his colostomy?

- Investigate common causes for fecal leakage and odor production.

- Analyze the client's normal dietary intake and consider foods that should be eliminated because they produce odors. Teach him how to clean his appliance and use bag deodorizers.

- Emphasize that his concerns and fears are normal and reassure him that he will adapt to his colostomy, its cares, and dietary regulation.

6. If you were the client, would it be best for you to take early retirement?

- Speculate about your feelings if you or a loved one had to have a colostomy.

- Identify your primary concerns upon your return to work. Consider the impact of colostomy care on maintenance of schedules, ability to work, and so on.

- Identify the client's strengths and limitations. List strengths that will allow him to successfully return to work. List limitations that could interfere with his ability to assume his normal work role.

7. What else may concern the client that he has not verbalized but frequently causes concern for people with colostomies?

   Place yourself in the client's situation. Identify other needs that have not been addressed, such as sexuality-related issues. Consider the physiological and psychological effects of the colostomy, such as feelings of inadequacy, body-image disturbance, fear of sexual rejection, and so on.

8. How will you know when the client is ready to assume responsibility for his colostomy?

   Identify data that suggest interest, curiosity, or acceptance. Consider client cues, such as asking questions, viewing the colostomy during care, asking for more information, reading the supplied brochures, and assuming responsibility for changing his colostomy bag.

9. What critical thinking attitudes and cognitive skills did you use to answer the questions pertaining to this case?

   Divergent thinking, reflection, intellectual empathy, and humility.

Community and Home Care Nursing
Congestive Heart Failure

The client is an 86-year-old widow who lives alone in a home about 25 miles from the nearest town. Her daughter lives 60 miles away and visits on weekends. The client no longer drives due to poor eyesight and, as a result, is homebound except for church on Sunday when she can get a ride. She describes herself as "very independent" and states that she hates being "fussed over."

The client enjoyed her usual good health until 2 months ago, when she was hospitalized with shortness of breath, fatigue, and peripheral edema, and diagnosed with congestive heart failure. Other medical diagnoses included arthritis, hypertension, and short-term memory loss. Her medications, upon release from the hospital, included 0.125 mg of Lanoxin every day, 20 mg of furosemide every day, 20 mEq of KCl twice a day, 325 mg of ASA every day, and 400 mg of Advil every 4 to 6 hours, as needed, for arthritis pain. The client has not kept her follow-up appointments at the local clinic and blames this on her lack of transportation.

On Wednesday morning, a neighbor called the clinic and reported that the client seemed ill. She refused to leave home because she feared being readmitted to the hospital, but she agreed to a home health care visit. Her physician asked the home health nurse to evaluate the client's physical status and her ability to care for herself.

Upon arrival at the client's home the nurse notes that the client is slow to answer the door and states, "I can't seem to wake up this morning." Her hair is uncombed and her clothes are rumpled, although the house is clean and well-ordered. The client is pleasant and cooperative but responds slowly, and her short-term memory loss is apparent.

The nurse notices that the client keeps her medications in a shoe box on the kitchen table. She admits to confusion about her medications and isn't sure if she's taking them correctly. She is unable to read the labels but does not want her daughter to know this. The nurse finds only three Lanoxin tablets in the bottle; there should be 12 remaining. The KCl bottle has too many pills. In addition, the client states that she stopped taking both these medications last week because they were making her sick.

The client is 5 ft, 4 in tall and weighs 120 lbs. Her blood pressure is 120/60, her heart rate is 54 beats per minute (bpm) and regular, her respiratory rate is 18 breaths per minute and regular, and her oral temperature is 98.6F. Upon auscultation, lung sounds are clear bilaterally. She has 1+ pedal edema, and complains of experiencing nausea, headache, poor appetite, fatigue, leg cramps, and drowsiness for at least the past week. In addition, she states that she has lost 3 lbs this week, and is short of breath when ambulating.

~~~~

1. What is your initial impression of the client?

   Analyze the subjective and objective data for patterns. Your initial impressions may include unreliable medication management, lack of social support systems, lack of transportation, fear of dependency, Lanoxin overdose with potential for digitalis toxicity, inadequate intake of potassium with potential for cardiac dysrhythmia development, and so on. Note data that support digitalis toxicity and hypokalemia.

2. What is the relationship between the client's symptoms and her current medication intake?

   • Investigate the effects and side effects of the client's current medications.

   • Speculate about the effect of underdosing or overdosing of these medications. Consider the relationship between overdosing of digitalis and digitalis toxicity, underdosing of potassium and hypokalemia, and underdosing of Lasix and exacerbation of clinical manifestations associated with congestive heart failure.

   • Review the complaints and symptoms of the client, including her nausea, headache, appetite, fatigue, leg cramps, and dyspnea.

3. What additional assessments need to be made?

- Review cardiac and pulmonary assessment parameters.

- Evaluate the necessity of a thorough respiratory system assessment given the client's diagnosis of congestive heart failure.

- Discuss the relationship between congestive heart failure and pulmonary edema. Consider other assessments that may be important, including the client's family or social support systems, her ability to obtain and prepare food, potential safety factors, and so on.

4. Of what significance is the client's heart rate?

- Consider possible causes of a heart rate below 60 bpm in an elderly client.

- Evaluate the client's medication intake and the effect of those medications on her cardiac status.

5. What nursing actions take priority in this case?

- Develop a problem list for the client.

- Prioritize the problems, noting those conditions that may be particularly harmful to the client, such as her inability to manage self-medication and the possibility of digitalis toxicity and potassium depletion. Consider appropriate actions, such as obtaining an electrocardiogram to detect cardiac abnormalities related to digitalis toxicity and drawing a blood sample to determine digitalis and potassium levels.

6. Should the client's family consider placing her in a long-term care facility?

- Identify the client's strengths and limitations. Consider the fact that she wants to remain independent and fears readmission to the hospital.

- Speculate about the advantages of institutionalization in light of her short-term memory loss. Consider alternatives to placing the client in a long-term care facility, such as assisted living or foster care.

7. How can you help the client keep track of her medication intake?

- Investigate the availability and usefulness of various devices designed to help people keep track of their medication schedules, such as pill containers that identify the week or month, containers that have alarms, or plastic pill baggies taped to a calendar.

- Weigh the advantages and disadvantages of these systems. Consider how you or your family members remember to take prescribed medications.

- Identify how mnemonic devices might be useful to someone with short-term memory loss.

8. How does the medication role of the home health nurse differ from that of the acute care nurse?

- Explore how medications are dispensed at home versus the acute care setting. Consider information that the home health nurse must teach that is unnecessary to convey while the client is hospitalized.

- Identify additional assessments that must be conducted at home that are not encountered in the acute care setting, such as compliance to a medication regimen.

9. What critical thinking skills did you use when addressing the problems in this case?

Divergent thinking, creativity, intellectual perseverance, humility, and so on.

Community and Home Care Nursing
Crisis Intervention

The client is a 20-year-old student who lives in the university dormitory. He tends to be a loner who does not make friends readily, even though he is frequently seen on campus and around the dormitory. On Wednesday, the hall monitor tells the residential advisor that he has not seen the client for a couple of days. The residential advisor knocks on the client's door several times but does not get a response. The door is locked.

Campus security is notified. When the security guard arrives, the residential advisor asks all of the students in the area to return to their rooms. The security guard unlocks the door and enters the room. They find the client sitting on the floor in the corner of the room. He is dirty and the room is a mess. There is a strong smell of urine.

When the security guard speaks to the client, he quietly tells the guard to leave or he will be sorry. The client looks away and refuses to answer any of the guard's questions. The university nurse is summoned to the room.

~ ~ ~ ~ ~

1. What safety considerations should the nurse weigh prior to speaking with the client?

   Research possible nursing actions for crisis intervention. Consider actions such as keeping the door to the room open; having a backup security guard nearby; using a controlled, soft tone of voice; knowing when backup assistance is needed; being alert for possible weapons in the room, and so forth.

2. What are some possible reasons for the client's reaction?

List possible reasons for the client's withdrawn behavior. Consider the possibility of excessive stress, psychotic reactions such as delusions or hallucinations, suicidal ideation, homicidal thoughts, a possible drug reaction, and so on.

3. What data are needed to support any of the previously mentioned possibilities?

- Review the data provided, clustering information into physical and psychosocial categories.

- Decide what further data are needed to support a conclusion for the client's behavior, such as suicidal thoughts, drug reaction, and so on. Consider the client's past medical history and information from his parents, roommate, classmates, and others. Consider the appearance of his room, noting the presence of alcohol, weapons, and other potentially dangerous items.

4. What interventions are most appropriate given the circumstances of the case?

- Review crisis intervention theory.

- Discuss how the theory applies in this case. Consider the need for the nurse to introduce herself or himself, express concern and offer help, have the security guard stay out of view, clear the area of students, ask the client for his impressions, and so on.

- Discuss the need for a plan of action in case the client refuses to leave his room voluntarily, stressing the value of encouraging cooperation before considering force.

5. How would you prioritize your interventions?

Using crisis intervention theory or another framework, prioritize the interventions you identified. Consider the need to maintain safety of both the nurse and the client.

6. What are the possible consequences to the client if you base your decisions on inadequate data?

   • Discuss how incorrect conclusions can lead to incorrect interventions. Consider how assumptions based on inadequate data can lead to prejudice.

   • Cite examples of other instances in which incorrect conclusions can compromise client care and safety or caregiver safety.

7. What attitude and cognitive critical thinking skills did you use to address this case?

   Faith in reason, creativity, reasoning, clarification, and so on.

Community and Home Care Nursing
Decubitus Ulcer

The client is an 89-year-old retired musician who suffers from dementia and prefers to stay in bed much of the time. He is being cared for by his daughter with whom he now lives. He was hospitalized for pneumonia and returned home after 7 days. The home health aide visits daily to assist with his care, and the home health nurse visits once a week.

Upon making a routine visit to the client, the home health nurse finds him lying quietly in bed. He is awake and able to briefly answer questions. His lungs are clear to auscultation and his respirations are nonlabored. His blood pressure is 110/72, his pulse is 80 beats per minute (bpm) and regular, his respirations are 18 breaths per minute and regular, and his oral temperature is 98.4F. His only medication is 500 mg of erythromycin 4 times a day to treat the pneumonia.

The nurse asks the client's daughter to help turn the client in order to complete the physical examination. They discover a 10-mm stage III decubitus ulcer on his sacral area. An ulcer was not noted in the hospital discharge orders, nor was the daughter aware of the ulcer. After discussing the problem with the client's physician, the nurse obtains aerobic and anaerobic wound cultures and applies a wet-to-moist normal saline dressing to the wound. After 72 hours, the wound cultures show no growth.

~~~~

1. What is your initial reaction to the client's home situation?

   • Consider data that influence first impressions or reactions, such as the presence of the pressure ulcer and the daughter's lack of awareness.

   • Assess the daughter's ability to care for her father, including her knowledge base and motivation level.

2. Why do you think the client developed a decubitus ulcer?

Review the data in this case, noting risk factors for pressure ulcer development, such as the client's age, nutritional status, inability to care for himself, recent hospitalization, and so on. Consider factors that promote ulcer formation, such as lack of activity, prolonged periods of bed rest, and shearing of linens.

3. What other data would be useful in deciding why the client developed a decubitus ulcer?

Consider your answers to the previous questions. Identify further data that are needed to determine the cause of the ulcer, such as the client's height and weight, length of time since his hospitalization, frequency of being turned throughout the day and night, and so on.

4. What is the significance of the cultures lack of growth?

Investigate the purposes of culturing a wound. Examine the reasons why cultures do show growth. Consider possibilities for the lack of growth in this case, such as absence of infection, improper culturing technique, and so on.

5. Why should you use wet-to-moist dressings on the client's wounds?

- Examine various methods of treating pressure ulcers, including wet-to-dry dressings.

- Review the concepts of tissue debridement and granulation.

- Discuss the benefits of using wet dressings to debride pressure ulcers.

- Discuss alternative treatments for pressure ulcers that may be as effective or more effective than wet-to-dry dressings.

6. What are the advantages of delaying judgment about the client's care until you have obtained all the facts?

   - Think about the consequences of drawing conclusions or making decisions on the basis of incorrect or insufficient data. Consider the potential for misjudging the daughter or home care aide regarding their care of the client.

   - Cite examples of instances in which forming premature conclusions was detrimental.

7. What critical thinking attitude and cognitive skills did you use to address this case?

   Basic support, clarification, reflection, faith in reason, and so on.

Community and Home Care Nursing
Fecal Impaction

The client is an 82-year-old man who has lived at home for several months following a cerebrovascular accident (CVA). A home health aide visits daily to bathe him and provide personal care, and a home health nurse visits every 2 weeks to oversee his care and monitor his indwelling catheter. Beyond these visits, his wife cares for him.

On Monday morning, the client's home health aide called the office and reported, "The client's wife says her husband hasn't had a bowel movement for about a week." The nurse contacts the client's physician and obtains an order for an extra nursing visit to check for a fecal impaction.

When the nurse approaches the client he states, "You've got to do something; my stomach is about to burst." He further complains of abdominal cramping and inability to have a bowel movement. The client's wife states, "I can't remember the last time he had a bowel movement, maybe a week or so ago." The nurse's rectal examination reveals a fecal impaction. She administers a Fleet enema, with poor results, and then removes the impacted stool manually. A second Fleet enema brings further relief, and the client tolerates the procedure well. The nurse explains to the client that he will need another enema later to completely remove the large amounts of impacted stool.

The nurse asks several questions to determine why the client became impacted. The answers reveal that he often misses his stool softener, drinks only small amounts of fluids, eats poorly, and does not like to get out of bed because of the difficulty it entails. The client's wife admits that she sometimes gives her husband mineral oil instead of using the stool softener.

The client's medical history includes hypertension and two transient ischemic attacks, followed by a left-sided CVA. As a result, he has right-sided hemiparesis, mild dysphasia, and dysphagia, making him dependent on others for most activities of daily living. He has a urinary catheter and has been evaluated for a feeding tube, which he does not want. His medications include 100 mg of Colace every day, one sustained-release capsule containing 120 mg of propranolol every day, 5 mg of Coumadin every day, and 50 mg of Zoloft at bedtime.

The client is a thin, serious-looking man who is alert and cooperative but in obvious discomfort. His blood pressure is 140/80, his heart rate is 74 beats per minute (bpm) and regular, his respirations are 16 breaths per minute and regular, and his oral temperature is 98.4F. The urinary catheter is patent with 200 mL of clear, dark-gold urine in the bag.

~~~~

1. What are the client's current priority nursing diagnoses?

   • Cluster available data, identifying cues to pertinent physical and psychosocial problems.

   • On the basis of your data clusters, prioritize the client's nursing diagnoses. Consider problems such as impaction and knowledge deficit.

   • Discuss how the wife's knowledge deficit may have caused her husband's impaction. Consider the value of addressing the client's impaction problem without resolving his knowledge deficit.

2. What effect do the client's medications have on his current condition?

   • Investigate the actual and potential adverse effects of the client's prescribed medications.

   • Identify medications that can produce constipation.

   • Discuss the need for increased fluid intake when taking any prescription or over-the-counter medications that decrease intestinal motility.

3. Which interventions are appropriate for this client?

   • Compare your interventions with suggested activities for the Nursing Interventions Classification (NIC) intervention of Constipation/impaction Management.

   • Discuss aspects of care that are missing, such as assessment of the client's dietary and fluid intake and client teaching regarding contributing factors to constipation, the importance of taking stool softeners as prescribed, and measures that prevent constipation.

4. What factors, other than his medications and improper use of his stool softener, may have contributed to the client's development of a fecal impaction?

   Discuss the need for a thorough assessment of the client's daily activities, diet, and fluid status. Consider factors such as decreased level of activity, inadequate fluid intake, and lack of adequate dietary fiber, as well as ignoring the urge to defecate and relying on laxatives rather than natural sources, such as prune juice, to eliminate constipation.

5. What activities can you suggest to the client's wife that will prevent the development of another fecal impaction?

   • Review the causes and warning signs of fecal impaction, such as hard stools, difficulty defecating, and frequent episodes of constipation.

   • Identify appropriate nursing activities, including anything that maintains or fosters peristalsis and regular bowel patterns, such as establishing a regular time each day to attempt defecation, drinking hot liquids, getting out of bed to assume a normal position for bowel movements, monitoring stools to detect when they are becoming too firm, and so on.

   • Discuss the importance of activity, diet, and fluid intake on maintaining the normal consistency of stools.

6. Are there any contraindications for using mineral oil to prevent the client's constipation?

   - Review the client's medications and investigate possible interactions between the prescribed drugs and mineral oil.

   - Identify mineral oil's effect on the absorption of anticoagulants such as Coumadin. Consider the relationship between the reliance on laxatives and development of constipation and fecal impaction.

7. What suggestions can you give the client and his wife regarding his difficulty ambulating to the toilet?

   Discuss community referrals or services that could assist the client, for example, a physical therapy consult to instruct the client and his wife about transfer techniques and make recommendations for medical equipment to assist the client with ambulation, such as a brace for his right leg and a walker.

8. What other clients are at risk for the development of fecal impaction?

   Consider all clients who have mobility problems, take medications that reduce intestinal motility, are unable to obtain or prepare high-fiber foods, are unable to drink an adequate amount of fluid, cannot communicate their needs, and so on. Research conditions such as multiple sclerosis, CVA, congestive heart failure, Alzheimer's disease, and chronic obstructive pulmonary disease.

9. What critical thinking attitudes and cognitive skills did you use to address this case?

   Divergent thinking, creativity, basic support, reflection, and so on.

Community and Home Care Nursing
Health Screening

The client is a 72-year-old widow who lives in a government-subsidized apartment complex for the elderly. She is generally described as a "talker" who enjoys participating in activities held at the complex. Today she decided to attend a mini health fair conducted by nursing students from a local nursing program.

At the first booth, the client learned that her blood pressure was 150/80, her heart rate was 78 beats per minute (bpm) and regular, her respiratory rate was 20 breaths per minute, her weight was 230 lbs, and her height was 5 ft, 3 in. She explained to the nursing student that she takes no prescribed or over-the-counter medications. A screening at the foot care booth revealed bilateral bunions. The booth workers attributed this condition on her poorly supported, thin canvas, slip-on shoes and suggested alternative footwear. With encouragement from a friend, the client decided to visit the breast cancer booth. While there, she was not as talkative as she was previously, but politely listened to the nursing student's explanation about the importance of monthly breast self-examinations. She accepted pamphlets on mammography and breast cancer, then leaned forward and whispered, "You know, I've got one of those lumps."

~~~~

1. What conclusions can you draw about the client on the basis of the data provided?

   • Discuss the obvious conclusions, such as breast cancer and hypertension.

   • Cluster data to determine related patterns.

   • Decide what further data are needed to support your conclusions.

2. What dilemma is presented by this case?

- Consider the need to refer the client for immediate evaluation without causing her to become overly anxious or fearful.

- Discuss the role of nursing students conducting health fairs and their responsibility to refer appropriate participants for further evaluation.

3. As a student nurse, what is your most appropriate response in this case?

- Discuss the need to obtain further data from the client, such as the name of her primary care provider, the date of her last physical examination, and so on.

- Discuss the importance of referring the client for immediate evaluation.

- With a classmate, role-play your response to the client.

4. Of what significance is the client's blood pressure?

- Review normal physical assessment parameters for the elderly.

- Research the pathophysiology of hypertension.

- Identify factors that place the client at increased risk for hypertension.

- Discuss the relationship between the client's weight and her blood pressure.

5. What attitude and cognitive critical thinking skills did you use to address this case?

Reasoning, divergent thinking, basic support, intellectual perseverance, and so on.

The client is a 72-year-old retired teacher who has type I (insulin-dependent) diabetes mellitus. The home health nurse visits every 2 weeks to fill her insulin syringes and check her general condition. When the nurse arrives at 11:00 AM, the client complains of nausea and states that she has vomited several times since breakfast. The nurse observes that the client is pale, her skin is cool and clammy, and her speech is slurred. The client says she took her insulin this morning and then ate breakfast as usual but thinks she vomited her breakfast. She checks her blood glucose every morning, but she didn't do so today because she felt too ill. Her normal blood glucose is 150 to 200 mg/dL.

The client's blood pressure is 88/50, her heart rate is 120 beats per minute (bpm) and weak and thready, her respirations are 28 breaths per minute and regular, and her oral temperature is 98.4 F. The nurse checks the client's blood glucose with a handheld monitoring device, which indicates a blood glucose level of 40 mg/dL.

~~~~

1. What do you think is happening to the client?

   • Cluster the data into related categories.

   • Identify problems suggested by the data clusters. Consider impending shock related to osmotic diuresis or insulin shock and the need for immediate intervention.

   • Decide if the data support diabetic coma or insulin shock.

   • Differentiate between the clinical manifestations of each.

2. Considering the assessment data, what should you do first?

- Review the significance of a blood glucose level of 40 mm/dL in a known diabetic patient.

- Discuss immediate measures that you can implement to increase blood glucose levels, such as eating candy or drinking orange juice.

- Discuss appropriate client care after such interventions have been implemented.

3. Evaluate the client's "normal" blood glucose levels.

- Research current literature about maintenance of blood glucose levels in diabetic patients.

- Discuss the relationship between chronically elevated blood glucose levels and the development of cardiac, renal, and vascular disease. Consider the need for lowering the client's blood glucose levels consistently.

4. What other data would be helpful when planning care for the client?

Consider obtaining information about her current medications, recent illnesses, dietary intake for the past several days, usual degree of blood glucose control, recent stressors, and so on.

5. What nursing interventions would be helpful after the client's blood glucose levels have returned to normal?

- Identify the client's strengths and limitations.

- Develop a problem list, noting problems that require immediate intervention.

- Identify nursing diagnoses that address each problem.

- Write nursing interventions specific to each nursing diagnosis. Use the Nursing Interventions Classification (NIC) to determine appropriate interventions.

6. How does type I diabetes mellitus differ from type II diabetes mellitus?

   Review the pathophysiology of diabetes mellitus, noting the differences between type I and type II, such as etiology, pathology, and clinical manifestations.

7. In this instance, why is it important to know which type of diabetes the client has?

   Review typical care of a client with diabetes. Note whether client care differs depending on the type of diabetes mellitus. Consider diet, medication therapies, and complications.

8. What critical thinking skills did you use to answer the questions pertaining to this case?

   Intellectual perseverance, clarification, basic support, reasoning, and so on.

Community and Home Care Nursing
Infected Foot Wound

The client is a 19-year-old student who lives with his mother in a mobile home. He is mildly retarded and attends special education classes for vocational training. The client is being treated for a deep wound to the plantar surface of his right foot, which occurred when he stepped on broken glass in the yard. The wound was sutured in the emergency department. The nurse there gave him and his mother supplies and taught them how to change the dressing daily. He received a tetanus injection and was placed on oral antibiotics for 10 days. Because of doubts about the client's home situation, the physician requested that a home health nurse visit the client twice a week to assess the wound.

Upon arrival, the nurse notes that the mobile home is cluttered, with uneaten food, clothing, and dirty dishes scattered around the rooms. There are no screens in the windows. The nurse finds the client sitting on the couch, watching cartoons on television. His personal hygiene is poor and the dressing on his right foot is loose and dirty. The nurse suspects that it is the same dressing he was given at the hospital 3 days earlier. Upon removing the dressing the nurse notes a foul odor, purulent drainage, edema, and redness surrounding the wound. The client admits to pain and tenderness, but he does not appear overly concerned. He states that he has been taking the medication ordered by the emergency department physician. The client's blood pressure is 140/70, his heart rate is 110 beats per minute (bpm) and regular, his respiratory rate is 18 breaths per minute and regular, and his oral temperature is 101.2F. The nurse obtains aerobic and anaerobic wound cultures, redresses the wound, and draws blood for a complete blood count (CBC).

~~~~

1. How do you feel about this situation?

   Consider how your biases regarding this client and his mother may influence your first impression. Assess your impressions pertaining to dirtiness, the condition of the home, the condition of the dressing and wound, and so on.

2. What data suggest that the client has a wound infection?

   - Review the process of inflammation and infection.

   - Discuss the local and systemic clinical manifestations of infection.

   - Compare your findings with the data about the client. Consider his complaints of pain and tenderness, his fever, and the appearance of the wound.

3. Why was it necessary to culture the client's wound?

   - Review the data about the appearance of the client's wound. Note clinical findings that support the presence of an infection.

   - Review implications for obtaining cultures, including the need to identify the presence and type of pathogens to determine what medications will be most effective in treating them.

4. What important data will the CBC provide?

   - Review the components of the CBC and normal findings.

   - On the basis of the client's assessment, speculate about information that the CBC will provide, such as increased white cell count, bacteremia, and so on.

5. How could this situation have been avoided?

   Discuss the benefit of a visit immediately following discharge to assess the home environment, the ability of the caregiver to assume responsibility for a mentally challenged individual, the financial resources of the mother, and so on. Assess the degree of teaching required for both the client and family prior to discharge.

6. What attitude and cognitive critical thinking skills did you use to answer the questions pertaining to this case?

   Intellectual humility, clarification, basic support, reasoning, and so on.

Community and Home Care Nursing
Medication Error

A 68-year-old woman who lives with her husband was recently hospitalized for osteomyelitis. She returned home with a central line for an additional 6 weeks of antibiotic therapy. With the help of her husband, the client self-administered vancomycin intravenously every day. The home health nurse was scheduled to visit 2 to 3 times a week to monitor the treatment.

The client's physician also ordered one tablet containing 1.0 mg of Coumadin daily to help keep the central line patent. When the client took the prescription to her pharmacy, the order was misread and she received 10 mg of Coumadin. During the initial visit, the client's home health nurse compared the medications in the home with the hospital orders and discovered the discrepancy. Fortunately, the client had only taken one dose from the new vial of Coumadin. The nurse immediately notified the physician and the pharmacy.

~~~~

1. How could this error have been avoided?

   - Discuss the faith that clients place in their pharmacists to accurately fill their prescriptions.

   - Discuss circumstances in which nurses have made medication errors similar to this pharmacist, for example, working with multiple distractions, misreading a label, and so on. Consider whether a pharmacist or technician filled the prescription and how this person's education can affect accuracy.

   - Discuss the need for clients to be taught how to read medication bottles and know the correct dose of their prescribed medications.

2. What do you need to teach the client?

   Consider teaching the client how to read medication labels, how to compare these labels with written instructions regarding her medications, and so on. Think of your own or your family members' prescribed medications and whether you or they carefully check labels for accuracy.

3. What are the possible consequences of the client taking too much Coumadin?

   • Review the actions and side effects of Coumadin. Consider the impact of one dose versus numerous doses.

   • Identify clinical manifestations of Coumadin overdose, such as bruising and bleeding.

4. Would this incident have been as likely if the client had been 28 years old as opposed to 68?

   • Consider whether you would note an incorrectly filled prescription.

   • Consider if any differences exist between a 28-year-old's and a 68-year-old's ability to read and understand medication labels.

   • Weigh the concerns of a 28-year-old versus those of an older adult.

   • Identify which person is more concerned with health issues. Consider whether client age influences a pharmacist's ability.

5. In your opinion, is it reasonable for this client to be able to manage her medication?

   • List the cognitive and functional abilities that are necessary in order to manage self-medication. Consider a person's age, eyesight, hearing, ability to remember, etc.

   • Suggest ways to help clients with managing their medications at home.

6. What critical thinking skills, attitude, and cognitive skills did you use to answer the questions pertaining to this case?

   Faith in reason, reflection, creativity, and so on.

Community and Home Care Nursing
Neighborhood Assessment

While driving to an appointment in an unfamiliar part of a large southern city, a public health nurse surveyed the neighborhood through the windshield. As he left the agency, he traveled on a raised thoroughfare. He noted debris along the cement barriers and recognized a government housing project noted for its high crime rate. As he approached his exit, he began to notice wood duplexes that he estimated were around 100 years old. In the first block a funeral home stood between a car repair shop and a fast-food restaurant. Several groups of men had gathered in front of a corner grocery store and adjacent bar. Several women who appeared to be teenagers were walking with baby strollers and small children. Numerous children rode by on bicycles.

In the next block a group of young men was sitting on the front porch of a house with boarded windows and graffiti-laden walls. An obvious statement on one of the walls read "RIP." As the nurse passed a neighborhood park, which was devoid of functional, safe playground equipment, he noticed an elderly woman sitting on a tree stump. Next to her was a grocery cart filled with pieces of cardboard, a broken chair, and a mop handle. A dress was drying on a nearby stump.

Upon return to his agency, the nurse reported his observations to his supervisor.

~ ~ ~ ~

1. What conclusions can you draw about this neighborhood on the basis of the data provided?

   - Consider the disarray of the neighborhood, possible lack of employment or activities, age and condition of the structures, and so on.

   - Assess the need to collect adequate facts before you draw conclusions that may be false or unsupported.

2. What further data are needed to support your conclusions?

   - Review your information.

   - Cluster data into related groups and identify patterns.

   - Determine what further facts are needed to validate your conclusions.

3. How can the nurse or agency address some of the potential problems noted in this neighborhood?

   - Identify possible neighborhood problems, such as teen pregnancies, gangs, poor housing conditions, homelessness, and so on.

   - Rate problems on the basis of their difficulty to address.

   - Identify which problems the community health nurse can effectively address.

   - Explore services available in your community.

   - Decide if any of those services would benefit this community.

4. What are your own biases about this neighborhood?

   - Analyze your reaction to this case.

   - Identify your feelings about the neighborhood.

   - Compare this neighborhood with your own. Consider whether you would be comfortable living in this neighborhood.

5. What attitude or cognitive critical thinking skills did you use to address this case?

   Intellectual humility, empathy, reasoning, clarification, among others.

Community and Home Care Nursing
Palliative Care

The client is a 58-year-old accountant. Last year he went to his family physician, at the insistence of his wife, with complaints of chronic cough, hoarseness, and difficulty breathing upon exertion. A computed tomography (CT) scan detected the presence of a tumor that was diagnosed as squamous cell carcinoma of the left superior lung lobe. Since diagnosis he has undergone a resection of the affected area of the lung and chemotherapy. Last month he learned that the cancer had metastasized to his liver and bones.

The client is married and has two adult daughters who are in frequent contact with their parents. His youngest daughter is pregnant with her first child. The client has smoked a half pack of cigarettes a day for 20 years. He considers that the damage is already done to his lungs, so he sees no reason to quit smoking now. He maintains that he is going to "die a happy man."

The client has recently returned home following radiation treatment to reduce the size of the remaining tumor, which proved to be ineffective. He requested that he be allowed to go home to die. His only medication is two 40 mg tablets of morphine sulfate every 4 hours and an additional 20 mg dose that he can take as needed. A nurse has been requested to visit the client at home to provide emotional support, monitor his pain status, and manage his symptoms.

Upon arriving at the client's house, the nurse notes that he is lying in bed. He appears thin and lethargic. The client is able to get out of bed slowly to use the commode, but his dyspnea increases with activity. The client is receiving oxygen through a nasal cannula. His oral temperature is 99.5F, his heart rate is 56 beats per minute (bpm) and regular, his respiratory rate is 32 breaths per minute and labored, and his blood pressure is 90/58. The client's wife states that her husband has vomited several times over the past 24 hours and is unable to keep down much more than a few sips of 7-Up. He is complaining of a great deal of pain. He turns toward the nurse and says, "I just want to die. This is becoming too difficult."

The client's wife and his daughters are very upset. The daughters maintain that their father is too young to die and feel that his judgment is being impaired by his pain medication. They want him returned to the hospital so that everything possible can be done for their father if he should go into cardiac arrest. The client's wife remains silent.

~~~~

1. What are the most pertinent issues in this case?

   Review the case, listing each possible issue. Consider the client's issues regarding the right to die and his competency, the family's issues of loss and grief, and the legal and moral issues of this case.

2. What roles, other than that of case manager, will the nurse play with the client and his family?

   - Review the roles of the home care nurse, such as advocate, mediator, counselor, and supporter.

   - Identify specific tasks performed within each of these categories. Consider your role in caring for the client's physical needs as well as his emotional needs.

3. Whose rights should take precedence?

   - Imagine what the client is experiencing. Imagine what the family members are experiencing.

   - From an emotional perspective, decide whose rights take precedence.

   - Discuss the client's legal rights in this situation.

4. Does the use of narcotic analgesics render the patient incompetent to make his own decisions?

   Review instances in which narcotic analgesics do render a person incompetent, for example, signing an operative permit after receiving preoperative medications. Compare that scenario with the client's situation. Discuss the rights of dying clients in making their own decisions.

5. If you were the client, what nursing activities might help reduce your discomfort other than giving medications?

   • Imagine yourself in pain.

   • Identify comfort measures that successfully reduce your pain.

   • Discuss the value of warm baths, music, warm blankets and clothes, positioning, dimmed lights, presence of family members, and so on.

6. How does palliative care differ from other forms of care?

   Define the term "palliative." Consider characteristics of palliative care that differ from other forms of care, such as curative or restorative. Identify instances in which palliative care is the preferred approach.

7. Do you think the client deserved his illness because he smoked for 20 years?

   • Examine your own biases for or against smoking.

   • Discuss your beliefs about whether people are responsible for their own actions, such as smoking, sedentary lifestyle, high-fat or fast-food diets, and so on.

   • Argue in favor of the client's continued smoking at this point in his life.

8. What attitude and cognitive critical thinking skills did you use to address this case?

Clarification, basic support, reasoning, intellectual integrity, and so on.

Community and Home Care Nursing
Parkinson's Disease

An 83-year-old homemaker cares for her 87-year-old husband who has end-stage Parkinson's disease. The couple has one son who lives in another state but visits twice each year. No other family members live nearby and the client's wife has isolated herself to care for her husband. During the past 6 weeks the client's condition has worsened, and he is now bedfast and aphasic. During a visit, the son became concerned about the condition of the home. He notified the family physician who subsequently requested the home health agency to evaluate the client's condition.

The nurse finds the client in an old-style hospital bed with an egg crate mattress. The client's wife, who is a small woman, states that she is unable to turn him without help. She is devoted to her husband and spends most of her time trying to get him to eat. She is frightened and anxious about his condition, but says that she did not know help was available.

Upon examination, the client's blood pressure is 110/60, his pulse is 88 beats per minute (bpm), his respirations are 16 breaths per minute with clear lung sounds, and his oral temperature is 98.8 F. He exhibits classic symptoms of Parkinson's disease, including resting tremors, fixed gaze, drooling, and rigid extremities. He is alert but unable to speak, and he does not respond to questions. His wife states that he eats pureed foods and has difficulty swallowing.

The client is incontinent and wears adult diapers. He is clean but has developed skin breakdown, with reddened and excoriated areas over his sacrum and hips bilaterally. He also has shallow ulcers on each heel and ecchymotic areas on his upper extremities.

~~~~

1. What data are most pertinent regarding the client's present health status?

   - Identify relevant data.

   - Group data into normal and abnormal physiological and psychosocial categories, for example, physical: vital signs, lung sounds, presence of ulcers and skin breakdown, bruising, and difficulty swallowing; psychosocial: the wife's inability to provide adequate physical care, the client's inability to communicate, and so on. Consider appropriate nursing diagnoses, such as Impaired Skin Integrity, Impaired Swallowing, Total Incontinence, and Caregiver Role Strain.

2. On the basis of your data, what may you conclude about the client's present status?

   Draw conclusions on the basis of each of the data clusters from question 1. Consider the client's potential for physical compromise, such as his risk for aspiration, malnutrition, decubitus ulcers, urinary tract infections, and related sepsis. Consider the client's potential for emotional compromise resulting from his inability to communicate and complete self-care deficit, and consider his wife's potential for caregiver fatigue.

3. How would you prioritize the client's health problems?

   Review the nursing diagnoses you identified in question 1. Use a theoretical framework, such as Gordon's Functional Health Patterns, to prioritize the client's problems and nursing diagnoses.

4. Why is caring for a client with Parkinson's disease particularly challenging?

   - Review the pathophysiology of Parkinson's disease. Note the progressive nature of the disease, the strengths and limitations of treatments, and common problems experienced by people with Parkinson's disease.

   - Compare the client's clinical manifestations with the textbook description of Parkinson's disease.

   - List conditions from your research of Parkinson's disease that present a challenge to nursing care.

5. What are some alternative care solutions for the client?

   Discuss various care facilities that are available in most communities, such as long-term care, skilled nursing facilities, home health care, and assisted living, that could assist the client's wife while offering appropriate care for the client. Consider how each service may benefit the client or exacerbate his problems.

6. What advantages may home care have over other options?

   - Discuss the advantages of home care for the client, such as living in a familiar environment, which reduces possible confusion, costs, and loneliness, and having greater contact with family members and pets.

   - Discuss the current trend toward greater family involvement in care and greater availability of nurses who have extensive expertise in caring for clients at home.

7. What can be done to reduce the strain being placed on the client's wife as the primary caregiver?

   - Discuss aspects of the diagnosis of Caregiver Role Strain defined by the North American Nursing Diagnosis Association (NANDA).

   - Research community services that may be available to assist with the client's care, such as meals-on-wheels. Consider involving neighbors or church members to help with cooking, cleaning, or allowing the client's wife to enjoy a day away from her responsibilities. Consider hiring home health aides or housekeepers.

   - Analyze whether the wife should continue to care for her husband at home.

8. What critical thinking attitudes and skills did you use to answer the questions pertaining to this case?

   Divergent thinking, clarification, creativity, intellectual humility, and so on.

Community and Home Care Nursing
Peripheral Vascular Disease

The client is a 38-year-old single mother who lives with her 19-year-old son in an inner-city apartment. She has a history of alcohol and drug abuse, although she denies recent use of either. She also has a history of peripheral vascular disease and was recently hospitalized for amputation of her left great toe. Although her treatment was successful and restored pulses to her left leg, the amputation site has been slow to heal. The client has orders for dressing changes twice a day to the open wound at the surgical site. However, she refuses to change her own dressings, so her physician ordered home health visits.

The client always wears a heavy stocking on her right foot and keeps it tucked under her while her dressing is being changed. She refuses to let the nurse examine the right foot, saying, "the doctor just saw it, and it's fine. It's only my left leg I have trouble with."

~~~~

1. What inferences can be drawn about the client's situation?

   - Cluster the data into physical and psychosocial categories.

   - Examine these categories and identify possible problems.

   - From those problems, make inferences about the client's reaction, such as fear of another lesion that may result in hospitalization and further surgery, fear of her inability to live independently, and so on.

   - Decide if your inferences are justified by the data provided.

2. How are peripheral vascular disease and tissue necrosis related?

- Review the pathophysiology of peripheral vascular disease, in particular the effect of altered tissue perfusion.

- Relate altered tissue perfusion to cellular death.

- Discuss reasons why people with altered tissue perfusion heal more slowly that those who do not have such alterations.

3. What consequences could occur if you abide by the client's wishes?

- Consider problems associated with peripheral vascular disease and the need to identify those problems.

- Identify possible consequences to ignoring such problems, including loss of toes, loss of a leg, localized infection, systemic infection, and so on.

- Consider problems that may be missed if assessments are not made.

4. Compare the responsibilities of the home health nurse to the acute care nurse when dealing with patients who do not wish to be examined.

Discuss client's expectations in the acute care setting, such as frequent assessment of skin, vital signs, heart sounds, and lung sounds. Consider how treatment in your own home may change your expectations of health care providers, the need to seek permission prior to performing assessments or treatments, and your role as a guest in the client's home.

5. What critical thinking attitudes and cognitive skills did you use to address the problems in this case?

Divergent thinking, reasoning, clarification, intellectual empathy, and so on.

Community and Home Care Nursing
Tuberculosis

The client is a 75-year-old widow who lives alone. Following the death of her husband 10 years ago, the client's son moved next door and checks on his mother frequently. Last winter the client developed pneumonia following a severe episode of respiratory influenza. She spent several weeks in the hospital receiving intravenous antibiotics and glucocorticoids. When her condition did not significantly improve, further diagnostic studies were performed, which resulted in the diagnosis of pulmonary tuberculosis. The client's only known contact with tuberculosis was her mother, who died when she was 9 years old. The client's physician placed her on antimicrobial therapy, referred her to the Public Health Department, and scheduled follow-up care for her by a home health nurse.

On the second visit following the client's release from the hospital, the nurse noted that the client was losing weight and appeared weak and fatigued compared to her earlier visit. From questioning the client, the nurse learned that the prescribed medications were making her feel sick, and she was becoming intolerant of food. The client was cooperative but stated that she "just can't tolerate the sight or smell of food."

~~~~

1. What other important data should you obtain from the client?

   Discuss the importance of ascertaining whether the client is complying with her medication regimen, the amount of weight the client has actually lost, the presence of mouth ulcers or sores that would inhibit her from eating, and so on.

2. How are tuberculosis chemotherapy and loss of appetite related?

Investigate the medications commonly used to treat active tuberculosis, such as rifampin, ethambutol, streptomycin, and INH. Note the physical effects and side effects of medications that may alter appetite.

3. Why was the client referred to the Public Health Department?

- Review diseases that must be reported to the Public Health Department.

- Discuss the ramifications of these diseases to the general population and the role the public health or home health nurse plays in protecting the safety of clients and others in the community.

4. How will the client's disease status affect her family members or close friends?

- Review the communicability of tuberculosis. Consider people most likely to have been exposed to the disease, such as family members and close friends.

- Review screening procedures for individuals exposed to active tuberculosis.

5. How could the client have tuberculosis today if her only exposure to the disease occured when she was a child?

- Review the pathophysiology of tuberculosis, including primary and postprimary disease.

- Discuss factors that can activate tuberculosis years after exposure, such as physical debilitation, use of steroid medications, chronic disease, and so on.

6. What nursing activities might be useful to prevent the client from losing any more weight?

- Consider interventions designed to facilitate the intake of food and drink, such as encouraging the use of dietary supplements, small frequent feedings, and foods the patient enjoys.

- Discuss the need for daily intake monitoring.

7. What is one of the most important home health functions when caring for a client with active tuberculosis, and why is it so important?

- Review your role in caring for clients with active tuberculosis, including ongoing assessments, client education, and so on. Consider the need to monitor patient compliance with the prescribed chemotherapy regimen.

- Discuss the consequences of failing to comply with treatment regimens, such as spread of the disease and medication resistance.

8. What attitude and cognitive critical thinking skills did you use to address this case?

Divergent thinking, clarification, basic support, intellectual humility, and so on.

Community and Home Care Nursing
Urinary Tract Infection

The client is an 84-year-old retired autoworker who has had two myocardial infarctions and coronary artery bypass surgery 2 years ago. His wife cares for him at home. The client has had numerous problems since his cardiac surgery. He does not eat well, and his fluid intake is less than 1000 mL per day. He has a history of urinary retention and requires the use of an indwelling urinary catheter. A home health care nurse visits him every 2 weeks.

During a routine morning visit, the nurse notices only 150 mL of urine in the urinary drainage bag. His wife states that she hasn't emptied the bag since last night around 6:00 PM. The client's urine is cloudy and dark gold with a strong odor. The nurse further observes a small amount of purulent drainage from the client's urethra. He complains of mild lower back pain, which he attributes to lying in bed too long. His blood pressure is 130/90, his heart rate is 98 beats per minute (bpm) and regular, his respiratory rate is 20 breaths per minute and regular, and his oral temperature is 100.8 F.

The nurse changes the client's urinary catheter and obtains a urine specimen. After calling the physician, she draws blood for a complete blood count (CBC) and differential count.

~~~~

1. What conclusions can you draw about the client's condition on the basis of the data provided?

    • Separate normal from abnormal data.

    • Cluster the information into related categories and analyze the facts for patterns.

    • Consider possible causes for the client's symptoms, such as a UTI, urinary retention, systemic infection, and sepsis.

    • Compare manifestations commonly associated with a UTI with the client's clinical manifestations.

2. Why does the client have an increased risk for developing a UTI?

- Review factors commonly associated with UTIs, such as decreased mobility, inadequate fluid intake, presence of an indwelling catheter, inadequate perineal care, and the aging process.

- Compare those factors with the data about the client.

3. What do you think the CBC and differential count will show?

- Review normal and abnormal parameters for CBCs and differentials. Note elevations associated with infection.

- Consider the likelihood of seeing an elevated white blood cell count with a shift to the left, indicating immature white blood cells.

4. What is the importance of performing a urine culture and sensitivity on the client's urine specimen?

- Discuss signs that indicate the need for a urine culture and sensitivity.

- Review the type of information gained from a culture and sensitivity.

- Consider the types of organisms that can cause UTIs and the medications recommended for treatment of UTIs.

5. What consequences may occur if a UTI remains undetected?

Review complications associated with UTIs, such as sepsis, pyelonephritis, kidney damage, and death, in addition to the discomforts of urinary frequency, burning, and fever.

6 What attitude and cognitive critical thinking skills did you use to answer the questions pertaining to this case?

Divergent thinking, reasoning, basic support, intellectual courage, and so on.

Maternal-Newborn Nursing

Maternal-Newborn Nursing
Adolescent Mother and Attachment Issues

The client is a gravida III, para I who delivered a 6-lb, 5-oz baby boy 12 hours ago. Her mother, who is divorced, is present. The client shows no interest in her newborn baby. The client's mother holds, feeds, and changes the baby when needed. When the nurse offers to show the client how to bathe the baby, the client waves her away saying, "Oh, Mom will take care of all that." The client's mother smiles meekly and responds, "I guess I'll have to take care of him when we go home anyway."

The client's two previous pregnancies were terminated by abortion. She is 16 years old and attends tenth grade. She has shown ambivalence toward this pregnancy since the beginning and continued it only at the insistence of her mother.

~~~~

1. What data support the nursing diagnosis of Risk for Altered Parent/Infant/Child Attachment?

   Group the data, noting information that suggests altered bonding between the client and her newborn. Consider the effect of the client's demeanor toward her baby and the impact of her reasons for continuing the pregnancy on her attachment to the infant. Speculate about the client's role in raising her son.

2. What can you do to promote the bonding process?

   Review the Nursing Interventions Classification (NIC) for attachment promotion. Consider discussing the client's reactions with her; persistently involving the client in the care of her infant, consulting with the client's mother about the importance of her daughter participating in the care of her infant, and so on.

3. What should you teach the client?

   Review general teaching parameters for all new mothers. Consider the client's maturational level and her probable lack of knowledge about self-care following delivery, birth control, the need to abstain from sexual relations until after her 6-week checkup, the need for postpartal follow-up, and so on.

4. How will you know if the client is receptive to learning about her infant?

   Discuss indications that the client is ready for teaching, such as asking questions, observing your interactions with the infant, and displaying certain facial expressions or gestures. Discuss the need to be aware of your own prejudices in this instance.

5. Why do you think the client's mother insisted that her daughter continue the pregnancy?

   List possible needs, desires, or concerns of the client's mother, such as her need to be needed, desire for another infant, concerns about the client's pattern of abortions, and so on. Consider the client's mother's potential concern regarding multiple abortions and the effects they may have on her daughter.

6. What biases do you have in this case?

   Decide if you have strong positive or negative feelings about any aspects of this case. As the nurse, consider how your feelings could impact the care you provide.

7. What critical thinking skills did you use to address this case?

   Divergent thinking, basic support, clarification, and intellectual humility.

Maternal-Newborn Nursing
Cesarean Birth and Recovery

The client is a 27-year-old woman who delivered an 8-lb, 12-oz baby boy less than an hour ago by cesarean due to a complete placenta previa. This is the client's first pregnancy, and she voiced disappointment about not being able to deliver vaginally as the nurse prepared her for surgery.

The client has a low transverse abdominal incision that is covered by a clean, dry dressing. Her vital signs are stable with a blood pressure of 129/84, a heart rate of 92 beats per minute (bpm), respirations of 28 breaths per minute, temperature of 98.8F. She is easily aroused and complains of pain when awake. Although she has briefly seen her infant, the client has not yet had an opportunity to hold him.

~~~~

1. Why does placenta previa necessitate cesarean delivery?

   Review the etiology, pathophysiology, and consequences to the mother and baby of placenta previa. Discuss the risk of maternal hemorrhage and the threat of interrupted oxygen supply to the fetus during vaginal delivery of a fetus with placenta previa.

2. What risks are involved with emergency cesarean delivery that are generally not present with scheduled cesarean delivery?

   Discuss the necessary preoperative preparation procedures for anyone undergoing surgery. Consider the need for prohibiting food and drink and preparing the client physically and psychologically. Identify the possible risks of performing surgery on a pregnant woman who may be physically exhausted and psychologically unprepared.

3. What are the advantages and disadvantages of a low transverse abdominal incision compared to the classic midline incision?

Review the two types of cesarean incisions. Compare the advantages and disadvantages of both types of incisions. Consider the position of the incisions, the amount of postoperative pain produced by each, the likelihood of incisional rupture in future pregnancies, blood loss, ease of suturing, risk for gastrointestinal complications, and risk for infection with either incision.

4. How will you know if the client is developing postoperative complications such as hemorrhage?

Review the pathophysiology and clinical manifestations of hemorrhage. Identify subjective and objective data that indicate hemorrhage and early hemorrhagic shock. Consider the client's vital signs, complaints of thirst, skin color, and other signs of complications.

5. How would you prioritize nursing diagnoses for the client?

Using the data about the client and your knowledge base regarding postoperative care of a woman undergoing cesarean birth, identify several pertinent nursing diagnoses. Review the defining characteristics of the diagnoses you selected to determine their appropriateness. Using a framework, such as the life-preservation framework, prioritize your nursing diagnoses. Discuss your rationale for prioritizing the diagnoses as you did.

6. How will your discharge teaching for this client differ from that of a woman who delivered vaginally?

Identify pertinent teaching that applies to any new mother. Using your knowledge base about postoperative care, identify additional teaching that is necessary for the woman undergoing cesarean birth. Compare teaching about episiotomy care with abdominal incision care, including their risk for infection and typical pain status.

7. What are the advantages of responding to the client's concerns about her delivery method in a therapeutic manner versus a reassuring manner?

   • Discuss the differences between a therapeutic and a reassuring response. Give an example of each.

   • Explain the advantages of focusing on the client's feelings, communicating to her that she has been heard, and communicating your willingness to listen.

8. What attitude and cognitive critical thinking skills did you use to address this case?

   Basic support, clarification, creativity, and so on.

Maternal-Newborn Nursing
Early Postpartum: Vaginal Birth

The client is a 30-year-old woman who is a gravida II para I. Six hours ago she delivered a 7-lb, 13-oz girl following 9 hours of labor. She received an epidural block but required no other medications during labor. Upon delivery, the client suffered a second-degree laceration despite an episiotomy that was performed. The infant's Apgar score was 8 at 1 minute and 9 at 5 minutes. The infant girl appeared healthy and cried vigorously. The client was excited about the delivery but stated, "Oh, I do wish it had been a boy." The client's partner, who attended the birth, assured her that a baby girl was fine and they could always try again.

The client is in her room with the new baby and her partner. She is attempting to breastfeed the infant. It is 4:00 PM. The client has been up and is voiding without difficulty. Her fundus is firm and at the umbilicus. She is experiencing a moderate amount of lochia, which is rubra in appearance. Her only medications include Tylenol No. 3 for pain and daily Colace for a stool softener. Her vital signs are normal, and she is expected to be discharged in the morning.

~~~~

1. What information suggests a potential problem and, therefore, requires further assessment?

   Review the data, noting information that is normal and abnormal. Consider both the client's physical and psychosocial status. Discuss the implications of her statement about the baby's gender. Decide what further assessments need to be made.

2. What factors influence the position of the fundus following delivery?

   Review and discuss fundal evolution following delivery. Compare the textbook picture of fundal recovery with the client's data. Consider factors that may influence fundal position, such as a full bladder, the presence of a hematoma, and so on.

3. What are the highest priorities when planning the client's care?

   Identify the primary needs of the postpartal mother, considering the length of her labor, her second-degree laceration, fatigue, her fundal position, and her initial reaction to the baby. Formulate plans directed at maintaining safety, enhancing comfort, relieving fatigue, and so forth.

4. How should the client's assessments change within the next 24 hours?

   Review the physiological changes that take place following delivery and note common time frames for such changes. Compare the client's present status with the condition that is expected 6 hours after delivery. Identify patterns to look for over the next 24 hours.

5. Compare the nutritional needs of the client with those of the nonlactating mother.

   Investigate the calories, protein, carbohydrate and fat intake needs of the lactating mother versus the nonlactating mother. Determine how many extra calories are expended through breastfeeding.

6. How will you know if the client is bonding with her baby?

   Identify signs that indicate maternal-newborn bonding and lack of bonding. Discuss the consequences of addressing a maternal-newborn bonding problem before adequate information has been gathered or evidence of non-bonding has been noted.

7. What critical thinking components did you use to address this case?

   Faith in reason, classification, basic support, and divergent thinking.

Maternal-Newborn Nursing
Ectopic Pregnancy

The client is a 26-year-old woman who is a gravida II, para I and was admitted to the obstetrics unit with complaints of dark-red vaginal bleeding that had occurred for about 2 hours. She is at 10 weeks' gestation and has been experiencing slight cramping on her left side intermittently for several weeks. The client has a history of urinary tract infections and was treated with ampicillin 2 weeks ago.

She lives with her husband and 3-year-old daughter in a house located near both of the couple's parents. The couple is excited about the pregnancy, and they are looking forward to having a sibling for their daughter.

An hour prior to admission, the client felt a sharp pain in her abdomen that she described as feeling "like something breaking loose." Within several minutes she began to feel dizzy and weak. The client called her husband who summoned an ambulance.

Upon admission, the client's blood pressure is 90/50, her heart rate is 120 beats per minute (bpm) and regular, respiratory rate is 24 breaths per minute and regular, and her oral temperature is 99.6F. Fetal heart tones are absent.

The client's diagnostic findings are as follows:

Ultrasound: positive for ruptured ectopic pregnancy

Hematology: Hgb 7.8 g/dL, Hct 28%

~ ~ ~ ~ ~

1. How should you prioritize your assessments to protect the client's safety?

   Review the pathophysiology of ectopic pregnancy. Note indications of tubal rupture, hemorrhage, and shock. Compare the client's clinical manifestations with those of tubular rupture, hemorrhage, and shock. Consider assessing the client's vital signs, abdomen, mental status, circulation, and so on.

2. How are the client's last set of vital signs significant considering her complaints?

Review the pathophysiology and corresponding clinical manifestations of hemorrhagic shock. Note the relationship between blood loss and the client's symptoms. Describe how the body compensates to maintain equilibrium during early shock.

3. Of what significance is the client's recent urinary tract infection?

Review the causes of urinary tract infections. Identify risk factors that may have predisposed the client to developing frequent urinary tract infections. Assess how significant the infection is to her pregnancy or current situation.

4. How may the client's loss be affecting her?

Review the objective and subjective data. Identify potential physical and psychological losses, including possible destruction of her fallopian tube and ovary, termination of a wanted pregnancy, diminished self-image, and so on.

5. If you were the client, how could your nurse best support you during this event?

• Prioritize the client's physical and psychological problems. Decide if her physical problems or psychological problems take precedence.

• Discuss interventions to address the client's concerns while providing physical care.

• Explain how anxiety can amplify the shock process.

• Identify the client's husband's needs. Discuss nursing activities to help him emotionally support his wife, while recognizing his need for similar support. Use Nursing Intervention Classification (NIC) to design a care plan that addresses the couple's physical and psychosocial problems.

6. Physiologically, what are the consequences of a fallopian tube or ovary loss if repair is not possible?

Review the normal physiology of ovulation. Discuss the theory that loss of a fallopian tube leaves a woman 50% fertile. Consider the probability of future pregnancies occurring when a fallopian tube is removed.

7. What are the advantages of using oral methotrexate therapy as a medical treatment choice for ectopic pregnancy? Why is methotrexate contraindicated in the client's case?

Research the use of methotrexate for treatment of ectopic pregnancy. Discuss how the medication attacks and destroys fast-growing cells. Discuss the criteria for methotrexate use. Review the client's data regarding ruptured tubal pregnancy.

8. What critical thinking skills did you use to answer the questions in this case?

Divergent thinking, creativity, faith in reason, and intellectual courage.

Maternal-Newborn Nursing
Gestational Diabetes

The client is a 32-year-old woman who is a gravida IV, para III and is at 32 weeks of gestation. She is 5 ft, 4 in tall and weighs 200 lbs. Upon her last visit to the nurse practitioner, the client learned that she has gestational diabetes. The practitioner referred her to diet counseling and placed her on an 1800-calorie American Dietary Association (ADA) diet.

During the past week the client's blood glucose levels have consistently stayed between 180 and 200 mg/dL. The client states, "I've been trying to stick to my diet, but it's really so hard because I'm around food all day." She works as a waitress in a local restaurant. The nurse has asked her to report to the outpatient diabetes clinic daily for the next week for insulin regulation and further dietary teaching.

~~~~~

1. Why is it important for the client to control her intake?

   Review the pathophysiology of gestational diabetes. Discuss the risks associated with obesity, pregnancy, and delivery. Also review the risks associated with gestational diabetes. Determine how complications are reduced by decreased weight and dietary control.

2. What can you do to help the client control her diet so that her blood glucose will be better controlled?

Consider how factors such as the client's age, obesity, diabetes, pregnancy, and constant exposure to food contribute to her eating problems. Think of techniques that help you control your own eating when consistently exposed to food. Consider whether those mechanisms might help the client. Review studies that demonstrate that eating frequently is more effective than skipping meals or snacks. Identify the best snacks for the client, and foods she should avoid.

3. Considering gestational diabetes is a temporary condition, why is the client being placed on insulin?

Review the pathophysiology of diabetes mellitus and the complications associated with poorly controlled blood glucose levels. Discuss the current theory regarding maintaining blood glucose levels within the normal range of 80 to 120 mg/dL for all diabetics. Investigate the benefits gained using insulin for gestational diabetes as opposed to relying on dietary control alone.

4. Explore your initial reaction to this case. What feelings did you identify that may reflect a bias?

Identify common biases held against obese people. Discuss whether such biases are based on facts or conjecture. Analyze the basis for most biases.

5. What effect do biases have on client care?

   Explain how unidentified prejudices may affect the manner in which nurses relate to clients. Identify other groups of people who have so called socially unacceptable conditions and consider methods to decrease discrimination against those individuals.

6. What critical thinking skills did you use to answer the questions pertaining to this case?

   Creativity, reflection, clarification, and intellectual empathy.

The client is a 28-year-old woman who is a gravida II, para I. She has been treated on an outpatient basis since her 16th week of gestation for elevated blood pressure. She is now at 34 weeks' gestation, and her blood pressure ranges from 180/90 to 190/100. The client's medical record states that she is normotensive when not pregnant. Her previous pregnancy was uneventful except for the last month, during which time she experienced mild hypertension that resolved with bed rest and antihypertensive medication.

The client has not experienced a reduction in blood pressure this time, however, in spite of bed rest and treatment with Aldomet twice a day. Consequently, her physician has admitted her to the hospital for magnesium sulfate therapy. The client has a supportive husband who accompanied her to the hospital. He voices his concerns about both the client and their fetus.

Not long after initiating the magnesium sulfate intravenous drip, the client calls the nurse to her bedside, stating, "I don't feel very well. I think something is wrong, nurse." Upon further questioning, the nurse learns that the client is experiencing nausea, malaise, right upper-quadrant tenderness, and epigastric pain.

When examining the client, the nurse notes that she is flushed and perspiring profusely, has 2+ pitting edema of both feet and ankles, facial edema, and obvious muscular weakness. Her blood pressure is 188/96, her heart rate is 120 beats per minute (bpm) and regular, her respiratory rate is 26 breaths per minute and regular, and her oral temperature is 99.2F. Fetal heart tones are present at 152 bpm.

The client's diagnostic findings are as follows:

Hematology: hemolysis of RBCs, thrombocytes 98,000/mm^3, platelets 96,000/mm^3

Chemistry profile: SGPT/ALT 29 U/L, SGOT/AST 25 U/L

~~~~

1. What can you infer from the data provided about the client?

   Review the client's history, physical assessment, and laboratory data. Cluster data into related categories according to body systems, health patterns, and so on. Draw conclusions about the client's problems on the basis of the data clusters.

2. What are the possible consequences to the client if you do not recognize the client's condition?

   Review the complications associated with the hemolysis, elevated liver enzymes, and low platelet count (HELLP) syndrome that occurs with preeclampsia. Consider possibilities such as microangiopathic hemolytic anemia, hemorrhage, detached retinas, subscapular liver hematoma, hyponatremia, hypoglycemia, and death.

3. What physiological changes are causing the symptoms experienced by the client?

   Review the pathophysiology of preeclampsia and the HELLP syndrome. Discuss the damage to blood cells as they pass through small, damaged blood vessels; release of liver enzymes from blood flow obstructed by fibrin deposits; epigastric pain related to liver distention; vascular damage related to vasospasms; development of platelet aggregation, and so on.

4. How would you prioritize nursing activities for the client at this time?

Review priority nursing activities for clients suffering from the HELLP syndrome. Consider appropriate assessments, supportive care, and activities to prevent complications. Discuss the need for vascular support, such as the administration of fresh frozen plasma or platelets or the infusion of intravenous glucose; the need to lower blood pressure and intraocular pressure; preparation of the client for immediate vaginal or cesarean delivery, and emotional support of both the client and her husband.

5. What other potential problems could occur that require monitoring?

Research possible complications related to hypertension, induced labor, and magnesium sulfate administration. Consider monitoring for changes in vital-sign patterns, client complaints such as nausea, vomiting, or headache; the development of seizures; signs of fetal distress; changes in urinary output, and so on.

6. Why would you treat pregnancy-induced hypertension with bed rest and Aldomet?

Review the pathophysiology of pregnancy-induced hypertension and the effects of increased blood pressure on the mother and fetus, such as its impact on placental exchange. Consider the rate at which sodium is excreted when a person is in the recumbent position, the relationship between sodium and water excretion, and the effect of reduced sodium and water on blood pressure. Review the effects of the medication Aldomet and identify mechanisms of action that result in reduced blood pressure.

7. What factors predispose a woman to develop the HELLP syndrome?

   Review the etiology of the HELLP syndrome. Discuss the problems associated with detecting a syndrome that has no known cause and occurs in both primigravidas and multigravidas. Consider the syndrome's association with preeclampsia.

8. What is the prognosis for both the client and her fetus?

   Review the complications that can result from the HELLP syndrome. Discuss the impact of each complication on the mother's recovery time. Discuss the impact and possible dangers related to early delivery of the fetus. Compare perinatal mortality rates associated with preeclampsia, eclampsia, and the HELLP syndrome.

9. What critical thinking skills did you use to answer the questions in this case?

   Divergent thinking, reasoning, clarification, and creativity.

Maternal-Newborn Nursing
Hyperemesis Gravidarum

The client is a 24-year-old woman who is at 14 weeks of gestation and is a gravida III, para I. She lives with her husband, who is her primary support system, and her 6-year-old daughter. The client is a sales clerk but works only during her daughter's school hours. She and her husband are excited about her pregnancy and looking forward to having another child. They are, however, concerned that she will not carry the pregnancy to term because of her history of spontaneous abortions.

The client has been nauseous throughout most of her pregnancy to date and has lost 10 lbs over the past 2 weeks. She sought the advice of her health care provider this morning because of her inability to tolerate food or fluids for the past 2 days. He decided to hospitalize her with the diagnosis of suspected hyperemesis gravidarum. The client retches often and is vomiting greenish liquid. She is on complete bed rest with orders to take nothing by mouth, and she is receiving an intravenous infusion of 5% dextrose in lactated Ringer's Solution with multivitamins. In addition, her physician has ordered compazine suppositories for her nausea and vomiting. Her visitors have been restricted to her parents since her husband is out of town.

When examined, the client is oriented but lethargic. Her skin lacks turgor, and her urine is dark and concentrated. Her breath has a fruity odor. Her lungs are clear to auscultation and her respiratory rate is 28 breaths per minute. Her pulse is 92 beats per minute (bpm) and regular, her blood pressure is 108/84, and her oral temperature is 99.8F. She is connected to a fetal monitor, which shows a regular fetal heart rate of 152 to 156 bpm, in the left lower quadrant.

The client's diagnostic findings are as follows:

Chemistry profile: Ca 4.0 mg/dL, Cl 94 mEq/L, PO 2.1 mg/dL, K 3.5 mEq/L, Na 125 mEq/L

Hematology: Hgb 15.8 g/dL, Hct 52%, WBC 6200, platelets 450,000/mm^3

~~~~

1. Which data are relevant to the client's physical status at this time?

Note normal and abnormal laboratory and physical assessment data. Cluster abnormal data into related categories on the basis of life-preservation or Maslow's criteria. Draw conclusions about the client's hydration and electrolyte status and her fruity breath odor. Compare the client's clinical manifestations with the common indicators of fluid volume deficit, electrolyte imbalance, acid-base imbalance, or metabolic acidosis.

2. What are the possible consequences to the client if the nurse does not recognize the significance of abnormal data?

Review normal serum electrolyte values and the implications of abnormal values. Note the client's laboratory values that are potentially dangerous, such as her serum potassium level. Discuss the effects of hyperkalemia, hypovolemia, or acidosis on the client and her fetus. Review factors that compromise early pregnancy or cause death of the fetus and mother.

3. If you were the client, how could the nurse best intervene to enhance your comfort?

Identify measures to decrease the client's nausea, such as requiring bed rest, moderately restricting oral fluids, offering small amounts of carbohydrates frequently, providing mild sedation, administering antiemetic medications, limiting visitors, and controlling smells. Consider how correcting fluid and electrolyte abnormalities will affect the client's comfort level. Explain how fear contributes to discomfort or pain.

4. If you were the nurse, which of your past experiences could influence your care of the client?

   Consider your own past experiences or those of previous clients that were similar to the client's situation such as illnesses that produced nausea or vomiting, fears about the outcome of an illness or operation, pregnancies that were particularly difficult, and so on.

5. Which other groups of clients have similar problems?

   Identify other diseases or conditions that produce nausea or vomiting, such as chemotherapy, anesthesia, gastroenteritis, or chronic renal failure. Discuss conditions that can result in hypovolemia, such as hemorrhage, osmotic diuresis, or burns. Consider clients who fear a loss, such as the loss or disfigurement of a body part, one's own life, or the life of a loved one.

6. What interventions are most appropriate for addressing the client's concerns about another spontaneous abortion?

   Consider using interventions such as active listening, anxiety reduction, or coping enhancement. Discuss the probability of losing a pregnancy due to hyperemesis gravidarum. Practice communicating with a person who is concerned about a loss. Identify effective strategies for conveying hope and concern. Use Nursing Intervention Classification (NIC) to help identify appropriate nursing interventions.

7. How does pregnancy contribute to hyperemesis gravidarum.

Review the pathophysiology of hyperemesis gravidarum. Discuss risk factors for the development of this condition. Identify physiologic changes caused by pregnancy that result in severe vomiting.

8. What critical thinking skills did you use to answer the questions in this case?

Reasoning, creativity, intellectual humility, intellectual empathy, and so on.

Maternal-Newborn Nursing
Induction of Labor

The client is a 24-year-old woman who is a primigravida and an uneventful pregnancy at 42 weeks of gestation and is being admitted to the labor unit from her physician's office for induction of labor. She has had good prenatal care. The client is well-prepared for the birth experience, and she is accompanied by her husband who is excited and supportive. Her two nonstress tests (NSTs) have been reactive, and a contraction stress test (CST) was negative. Upon examination, the nurse notes that the client's embryonic membranes are intact and her cervix is soft, thick, and dilated to 1 cm. Her Bishop score is 8.

The client's physician orders continuous fetal monitoring with a 15-minute baseline followed by an intravenous (IV) infusion of Pitocin. The nurse initiates the IV infusion of 10 mL of Pitocin in 1000mL of lactated Ringer's solution through an infusion pump at 0.5 mU per minute. Since uterine contractions occurred within 15 minutes, the nurse increased the infusion to 1 mU per minute. Following a 2-hour period of induction, the client's contractions are occurring every 3 minutes and lasting between 60 and 70 seconds.

~~~~

1. On the basis of the client's data, what could happen if the physician had decided not to induce her labor?

   Review the primary indicators for labor induction. Compare the client's data with the textbook indicators for labor induction. Consider the length of her pregnancy and the risk to the fetus of remaining in utero. Discuss the effects of post-term pregnancy on the fetus.

2. What conditions must be met before the client's labor can be induced?

Review the criteria for labor induction. Consider the fetal lie and presentation, viability, cervical readiness, absence of cephalopelvic disproportion (CPD), and so on.

3. How do NSTs and CSTs differ?

Explain the meaning of NST and CST. Investigate the reasons for performing a CST or NST. Explain how the tests differ and describe the information provided by each test. Discuss the difference between a positive and negative CST.

4. What is the significance of the client's Bishop score?

Review the Bishop method of scoring that determines a client's readiness for elective induction. Explain each of the categories addressed by the score and interpret the client's score.

5. Why is it essential to administer Pitocin by infusion pump rather than by gravity?

Investigate the actions and side effects of the medication Pitocin. Consider the possibility of serious side effects, such as extreme hypotension, fetal death, and uterine rupture if the medication dosage produces excessive uterine contraction. Discuss the risks involved with administering Pitocin too rapidly.

6. Why was the client's Pitocin infusion started at 0.5 mU/min and advanced at 15-minute intervals?

Discuss the need to administer only enough medication to initiate and maintain uterine contractions. Identify the dosage at which most women respond to Pitocin. Discuss the need to avoid tetanic uterine contractions related to excessive Pitocin administration.

7. How will the nurse know when to stop increasing the Pitocin dosage?

On the basis of your research about the effects of Pitocin, identify assessment findings that indicate the ideal infusion rate has been reached. Consider both the frequency and duration of contractions.

8. Which conditions would necessitate discontinuing a Pitocin infusion?

On the basis of your research of the medication Pitocin, list complications that necessitate discontinuing the infusion. Consider effects such as alterations in fetal heart rate, including tachycardia or bradycardia, persistent late decelerations, or prolonged variable decelerations; contractions occurring more frequently than every 2 minutes and lasting more than 90 seconds, and so on.

9. How should you prioritize nursing diagnoses for the client and her fetus during labor induction?

Cluster subjective and objective data into related categories. Identify nursing diagnoses on the basis of your data clusters. Using the life-preservation framework or another framework, prioritize your identified nursing diagnoses.

10. What impact may nursing actions concerning the client's labor induction have on the outcome of her birth process?

   List and prioritize nursing actions related to the client's Pitocin infusion. Discuss consequences of Pitocin infusion that can occur if you do not assess and monitor the medication's administration appropriately.

11. How does induction differ from augmentation of labor?

   Define the terms "induction" and "augmentation." Review the differences in medication dosages, monitoring, contraindication, and procedures required for both induction and augmentation.

12. What attitude and cognitive critical thinking skills did you use to address this case?

   Basic support, clarification, reasoning, divergent thinking, and so on.

The client is a 27-year-old mother of one who gave birth to twin girls approximately 10 hours ago. The client and her partner were initially distraught when they learned that she was carrying more than one fetus because they had not planned to have more than two children. However, as time passed, they became accustomed to the idea and, by the end of the 7th month of pregnancy, were looking forward to their anticipated twins.

The client was in labor for 6 hours. Following vaginal birth of the first infant, a cesarean was performed to deliver the second infant due to premature placental detachment. The first infant weighed 5 lbs, 1 oz and had an initial Apgar score of 9. The second infant weighed 4 lbs, 4 oz, with an initial Apgar score of 7. Both infants were placed in warmers and monitored until they were stable. Neither infant is exhibiting signs of respiratory distress even though they are small for their gestational age of 38 weeks.

The client is now recovering. Her vital signs are stable, and her dressing is dry and intact. She is fatigued and sleepy but eager to hold and care for her infants.

~~~~

1. Why are multiple gestations considered high-risk pregnancies?

   Consider the physiological and psychological adjustments that a woman experiences during pregnancy, as well as the potential complications she may endure. Compare such adjustments for a woman carrying one fetus with those of a woman carrying more than one fetus. Explain why the woman carrying more than one fetus is more susceptible to pregnancy-induced hypertension, hydramnios, placenta previa, anemia, postpartal bleeding, and premature delivery. Consider the psychological impact of becoming the mother of two (or more) children versus the mother of one.

2. What were priority nursing diagnoses for the client during her pregnancy?

Select appropriate nursing diagnoses for a client with a multiple gestation. Compare the client's data with the defining characteristics of the nursing diagnoses you selected. Decide if the diagnoses are most appropriate for this client. Consider nursing diagnoses that address increased fatigue, risk for parental role conflict, fear related to her own health or that of her babies, and so on. Prioritize your nursing diagnoses on the basis of the life-preservation framework or another theory.

3. How does the client's birth process compare with that of a woman delivering one fetus?

Investigate the delivery needs of a woman with a multiple gestation. Consider the need for additional personnel to attend to possibly immature infants, the woman's fears and excitement, the possible need for a cesarean birth to decrease the risk to the second fetus, and so on. Compare the stages of labor for a woman with a single gestation to that of a woman with a multiple gestation. Compare their risks for complications, such as cord prolapse, uterine dysfunction, premature placental separation after delivery of the first infant, inappropriate presentation for vaginal delivery, and so on.

4. How will the client's nursing care differ now that she is in the immediate postpartum period?

Review the care of a client during the immediate postpartum period. List nursing diagnoses pertaining to this time period. Prioritize your nursing diagnoses in the same manner as you did for question number 2. Compare your pre- and postdelivery nursing diagnoses for similarities and differences.

5. Why is it especially important to maintain the newborns' temperature within a normal range since they were born prematurely?

Compare the thermoregulatory mechanisms of premature infants with those of term infants. Explain why premature infants are at a greater risk for temperature imbalances than term infants. Consider premature infants' decreased subcutaneous tissue, need for increased calories, increased oxygen use, and risk for respiratory distress.

6. How will having two versus one infant to care for affect the client's recovery?

Discuss the increased energy needs of the mother who must provide for two infants. Consider her nutritional needs, fatigue, pain status, incision, and so on.

7. If you were the client, what concerns might you have about caring for twins?

Reflect on your own experiences as a parent caring for children, as a sibling caring for younger brothers and sisters, or as baby-sitter caring for one or more children. Identify pleasurable aspects versus frustrating or energy-draining aspects. Identify how your concerns in those situations may be similar to the client's concerns.

8. What attitude and cognitive critical thinking skills did you use to address this case?

Divergent thinking, reflection, clarification, intellectual empathy, and so on.

Maternal-Newborn Nursing
Postpartum Depression

The client is a 19-year-old woman who returned home from the hospital yesterday with her newborn baby boy who is now 2 days old. The baby weighed 7 lbs, 1 oz at birth. His Apgar scores were 8 and 10. The client had a 12-hour labor and an uncomplicated vaginal delivery. During her admission to the hospital. The client decided to breastfeed and did well with the support and encouragement from her nurses. She was attentive to all teaching while in the hospital, but she frequently voiced concern about having to care for her newborn by herself. Because of a recent move, the client has few friends and no family members within the area who can offer emotional support or education regarding her newborn. Neither her parents nor her husband's parents are able to visit or offer assistance at this time. The client works long hours as manager of a fast-food restaurant and will only be available at night to help care for the baby.

The client's health insurance carrier allows for a home health nurse visit within the first week following hospital discharge; therefore, a nurse has been assigned to visit the client at home. Upon arrival at the client's home on her fourth postpartum day, the nurse notes that the apartment is cluttered and needs to be cleaned. The client appears disheveled and is sobbing. She states that she hasn't slept since coming home, she feels exhausted, and she can't take it anymore. She adds that the baby has finally stopped crying, for which she is relieved and grateful. The client states that if she had known that motherhood was going to be this difficult, she would never have had the baby. She feels she is a poor mother and incapable of caring for the baby.

The nurse notes that the client is pale but her vital signs are stable. She states that she passed a large clot yesterday but her drainage is decreasing. Her fundus has receded to approximately 3 cm above the pubic bone. She adds that she has little appetite and has had two episodes of diarrhea during the past day. She further states that she misses her family and friends.

The baby, who is now 4 days old, is in a small room off the client's bedroom in a crib. The client reluctantly allows the nurse to examine the baby, stating that she fears he will awaken. The nurse notes that the baby has excoriated buttocks, his skin is dry, and he is lying quietly in bed. The client states that she has tried to breastfeed him, but he keeps falling asleep. His rectal temperature is 102F, his apical heart rate is 180 beats per minute (bpm), and his respirations are 45 breaths per minute. His sclera are yellowish in color, and his fontanelles are slightly sunken. He weighs 6 lbs, a decrease of 17 oz from his hospital discharge weight.

~~~~

1. What inferences can you draw about the client's mental and emotional status?

   Cluster the subjective and objective data into related categories. On the basis of your data clusters, identify actual and potential problems. Consider the client's physical symptoms of fatigue, loss of appetite, diarrhea, and so on. Consider her psychosocial symptoms, such as feeling inadequate, wanting to cry, and missing her family and friends.

2. How are childbirth and postpartal depression related?

   Research the topic of postpartal depression. Explain the client's behavior on the basis of your findings. Discuss the hormonal shifts that occur following childbirth and the effect of those shifts on the client's mood.

3. At what point can postpartum depression become postpartum psychosis?

   Research the condition of postpartum psychosis. Compare the clinical manifestations of postpartum depression with postpartum psychosis. Consider the time at which both conditions may occur and the length of time they typically persist.

4. What can you infer about the newborn's physical status?

Describe the normal physical findings for a 4-day-old infant. Compare the client's newborn data with that of a normal newborn. Decide which data are abnormal and what the abnormal data imply about the newborn's status. Consider the newborn's weight, sunken fontanelles, lethargy, temperature, and so on.

5. Considering the assessment data on both the client and her newborn, what should you do first?

Review the significance of the newborn's physical findings. Research the importance of adequate fluid balance in a newborn. Using the life-preservation framework or another vehicle, prioritize both the needs of the client and her newborn. Decide which action to take first on the basis of your prioritization.

6. What is the most likely prognosis for the client given your understanding of postpartum depression?

On the basis of your research on postpartum depression and the client's current living situation, predict the outcome of the client's depression. Identify factors that can help clients overcome postpartum depression or perpetuate the condition. Discuss the need for immediate intervention to increase her chances for a full recovery.

7. What attitude and cognitive critical thinking skills did you use to address this case?

Divergent thinking, reasoning, clarification, basic support.

Maternal-Newborn Nursing
Primigravida Labor

The client is a 28-year-old woman who is a gravida I, para 0, at 40 weeks gestation. This morning she noticed mild contractions, which steadily increased in strength and duration. When the contractions were occurring every 7 to 10 minutes and becoming uncomfortable, the client asked her partner to return home. She then consulted with her nurse practitioner who suggested she remain at home until her contractions were about 5 to 6 minutes apart. Six hours later, the client reported to her birthing facility.

Upon assessment, the nurse notes that the client's contractions are 4 to 5 minutes apart, moderately strong, and approximately 50-seconds long. Vaginal examination reveals cervical dilation of 3 cm, 75% effacement, and -3 station. Her embryonic membranes are intact. The client and her partner are excited, although the client appears tired and groans with the contractions. She states, "I'll be glad when this is over; I don't think I can stand much more."

~~~~

1. Why did the nurse practitioner suggest that the client wait a while longer before reporting to the birthing facility?

   Review the normal labor process. Examine the differences in progression of labor between primigravidas and multiparas. Examine the advantages and disadvantages of remaining at home during early labor.

2. What can you infer about the client's assessment findings?

Identify physical examination parameters for the laboring client. Review the purpose of the vaginal examination and information that is obtained from it. Compare the client's findings with the textbook picture of the laboring client. Draw conclusions about the client's condition on the basis of the available data, including her stage of labor, progression, and so on.

3. What other data should you obtain about the client and her fetus?

Decide what other data is needed, such as the fetal heart rate, the client's obstetric history, her contraction pattern at home, the time that labor started, the presence of bleeding, the client's current medications, any allergies, and so on.

4. What conditions will you monitor for during the client's labor to ensure they are within specified parameters?

Define the terms "effacement", "dilation", and "station". Review monitoring parameters for the laboring patient, including those for fetal heart rate and pattern; frequency, intensity, and duration of contractions; degree of cervical dilation, effacement, and station; membrane status; pelvic status, and so on.

5. How will you know when the client needs pain intervention?

Discuss factors that influence the amount of pain a woman experiences during labor, such as preparation for and expectations of labor, perception of pain, length of labor, fetal position, availability of a support person or people, fear, anxiety, and so on. Identify data that indicate the presence of pain, such as certain statements, crying, increased heart rate, difficulty listening, and decreased ability to follow instructions.

6. In what ways can a support person influence the labor experienced by a woman?

Consider the relationship of the support person to the laboring woman. Discuss how the support person's fear or anxiety can influence the laboring woman's fear and anxiety. Discuss the benefit of having a "coach" if the laboring woman loses her ability to use controlled breathing, and other pain-reduction techniques.

7. Compare the client's reaction to labor with that of a multipara experiencing labor.

Discuss the advantages and disadvantages of prior experience with labor and delivery. Determine whether clients have the same experience with each subsequent labor and delivery. Discuss the impact of past experiences on present situations.

8. What critical thinking skills did you use to address the questions in this case?

Reasoning, creativity, clarification, basic support.

Maternal-Newborn Nursing
Puerperal Eclampsia

The client is an 22-year-old woman who is a gravida I, Para I. She experienced an uneventful pregnancy except for mild hypertension that did not require treatment. The client delivered an 8-lb, 1-oz baby boy vaginally 12 hours ago. Six hours after delivery her blood pressure was 110/68, her heart rate was 74 beats per minute (bpm) and regular, her respiratory rate was 12 breaths per minute and regular, and her oral temperature was 99.0 F. The client was up and about in her room. She and her husband were caring for the baby, and they were receiving visitors.

The client's husband, with a panicked look on his face, summons the nurse to the client's room, stating that the client suddenly gasped, grabbed her chest, and collapsed to the bed. The nurse quickly recognizes that the client is having an eclamptic seizure. The client's blood pressure is 190/110.

~~~~

1. What immediate actions need to be taken by the nurse?

   Review care of the client with preeclampsia, eclampsia, and seizures. Consider safety measures for the client and initiation of treatment to control seizures and decrease her blood pressure, such as fluid support and magnesium sulfate therapy. Identify priority assessments for the client.

2. Could this problem have been anticipated and thus avoided?

   Review the pathological events occurring with eclampsia, noting clinical manifestations that may forewarn you of its appearance. Discuss the relationship between pregnancy-induced hypertension and postbirth eclampsia.

3. What further data was needed in order to anticipate the preeclamptic state?

Carefully review all data pertaining to the client's physical status. Decide what data could have helped the nurse anticipate the client's seizure. On the basis of your research, cite nursing activities designed to prevent or detect eclampsia.

4. What precautions should the nurse take when administering magnesium sulfate to an eclamptic client?

Research the medication magnesium sulfate and the implications for its use as a treatment for eclampsia. Note both actions and adverse reactions of magnesium sulfate. Identify assessments and related parameters that need to be monitored to evaluate the effectiveness of the medication and indicate that side effects are occurring.

5. How will caring for the client help the nurse care for other patients who experience seizures?

Identify other clients who are at risk for seizures, such as those with epilepsy, a brain injury, and hypertension. Compare the care of these individuals with that of the client, identifying ways in which these clients are similar or different.

6. What critical thinking skills did you use to address this case?

Clarification, divergent thinking, reasoning, and basic support.

Maternal-Newborn Nursing
Teenage Pregnancy and Premature Labor

The client is a 16-year-old sophomore in high school. She is single and lives with her parents. The client is at 32 weeks of gestation with her first pregnancy. She had been experiencing lower back pain and slight abdominal cramping for 6 hours prior to coming to the hospital. Her vaginal examination reveals that she is 0-cm dilated and her cervix is thick and high. The fetal monitor shows mild contractions every 5 to 6 minutes and a fetal heart rate varying between 142 and 150 beats per minute (bpm). The client wants to have the baby now, stating, "I'm tired of this and want to get it over with. I've heard that lots of times premature babies do just fine." The client's parents and her 18-year-old boyfriend are at her bedside.

~~~~~

1. What can you deduce about the client's physical and psychological status?

   Identify data that are most relevant to the client's situation, including the client's age, maturity, support systems, emotional reaction to premature labor, and so on. Note both subjective and objective data. Cluster the data into physical and psychosocial problems. Make deductions on the basis of your data clusters, such as the client may not have enough information about the consequences of premature birth.

2. What additional data would further support your deductions?

   Review your deductions about the client's condition. Decide which questions or physical assessments are necessary to gain more information. Identify data that should be obtained from the client versus her parents, such as her knowledge of prenatal care, interest in prenatal classes, view of parental support, and so on.

3. How do the client's maturational needs differ from those of a woman in her late 20s or early 30s?

   Review the developmental tasks of the average adolescent, such as establishing self-worth and lasting relationships, becoming emancipated from parents, or choosing a vocation. Compare an adolescent's developmental stage with that of a woman in her early 30s. Discuss how the client's developmental needs may be positively or adversely affected by motherhood.

4. What is the significance of the client's statement about premature babies?

   Discuss whether this statement reflects the client's needs rather than those of her fetus. Consider factors that may have contributed to this statement, such as her possible lack of knowledge about the effects of premature birth on her baby, the permanency of having a child, and so on.

5. If you taught the client about the dangers of premature delivery at this time, how effective would such information be?

   Determine which teaching is essential while the client is hospitalized. Consider the client's ability to listen and understand while she is experiencing discomfort. Identify alternative methods of addressing the client's desire to have her pregnancy completed, such as focusing on her own health and readiness to experience labor and delivery as opposed to the infant's condition.

6. What biases, if any, do you hold about adolescent pregnancy? How may biases influence the care rendered to pregnant adolescents?

   Examine your own feelings about teenagers becoming pregnant and their ability to assume the mothering role. Speculate about your ability to care for a pregnant adolescent considering your personal biases.

7. How is the pregnant adolescent similar to the elderly primigravida?

   Review the risks associated with adolescent pregnancy and those associated with delaying pregnancy until the late 30s or early 40s. Explore the concept of high-risk pregnancy. Compare the risks associated with adolescent pregnancy to those of pregnancy later in life. Consider role changes required for both conditions. Note similarities and differences.

8. What critical thinking skills did you use to answer the questions pertaining to this case?

   Base support, intellectual integrity, clarification, and so on.

Maternal-Newborn Nursing
Uterine Tear

The client is a 39-year-old woman who is a gravida IV, para III, at 38 weeks' gestation. She reported to the labor and delivery unit complaining of uterine contractions. In 1 week, she is scheduled for an elective cesarean delivery. She states that she has been having lower pelvic pressure and mild contractions every 5 to 10 minutes, lasting 30 to 50 seconds. She called her obstetrician who advised her to go to the labor unit to be checked.

The client has three children, the last one of which was delivered by cesarean after the client's labor failed to progress. The section required a vertical abdominal and a vertical uterine incision, which required a ventral repair last year. When she was 8 weeks pregnant, she visited her present obstetrician who apprised her of the risks of her pregnancy.

The client's diagnostic findings on admission are as follows:

Hematology: Hgb 11.5 g/dL, Hct 43%

Upon examining the client, the nurse notes an indentation across her abdomen, abdominal rigidity, absence of vaginal bleeding, and no cervical dilation. Strong uterine contractions are occurring every 5 to 10 minutes. The client's blood pressure is 106/70, her heart rate is 100 beats per minute (bpm) and regular, and her respiratory rate is 28 breaths per minute and regular. Fetal heart tones are 146 bpm and regular; fetal monitoring shows no evidence of fetal distress. The client's husband is at her bedside.

As the nurse continues her assessment, the client suddenly complains of severe pain during a contraction. Within minutes the client's skin is cold and clammy, her heart rate is up to 120 bpm, her respirations are rapid and shallow, and her blood pressure drops to 100/76. The indentation across the client's abdomen is pronounced and contractions have ceased. The monitor indicates fetal distress. The nurse prepares the client for immediate cesarean delivery.

~~~~

1. What can be inferred from the client's admission data and present physical status?

   Analyze the client's data for evidence of a uterine tear. Discuss the relevance of the abdominal indentation, strong uterine contractions without cervical dilation, absence of vaginal bleeding, and so on. Consider the significance of fetal distress. Examine the relationship between blood loss and fetal distress.

2. Of what significance is the client's increased heart rate; drop in blood pressure; and cold, clammy skin?

   Review the clinical manifestations of hemorrhagic shock. Compare the signs of shock with the client's signs and symptoms. Discuss the structure of the uterus, its vascularity, and the degree of bleeding that can occur with uterine tears or rupture.

3. What are the possible consequences of uterine tear to the client and her fetus?

   Review the morbidity and mortality rates for uterine tear. Discuss the possibility of sterilization, death of the fetus, death of the mother, or death of both resulting from a uterine tear. Consider the psychological impact of the loss of child-bearing ability, loss of the fetus, or loss of a wife and mother.

4. What nursing actions should take precedence in this situation?

   Discuss the need for emergency nursing and medical interventions. Review protocols for hemorrhagic shock. Identify priority nursing actions for uterine tear, such as performing an accurate assessment; initiating emergency measures; providing close, continued monitoring; and preparing the client for an emergency laparotomy. Examine medical interventions, such as initiating fluid resuscitation, administering oxytocin to stimulate uterine contractions and control bleeding, and so forth.

5. What additional information, if obtained upon admission, may have indicated the seriousness of the client's condition?

   Discuss risk factors associated with uterine tear, such as previous cesarean section, ventral repair, and so on. Review the pathophysiology of uterine tear and associated clinical manifestations. Compare the client's data with clinical manifestations associated with uterine tear.

6. If you were the client, how could the nurse best support you emotionally as well as physically?

   Recall instances in which you thought your life was being threatened. Identify actions by other people that helped you feel safe and identify actions that escalated your fears. Discuss the need for implementing emergency measures in a calm and reassuring manner. Decide how your past experiences could help you render effective care to the client.

7. How can the nurse best support the client's husband while the client is being prepared for emergency surgery?

   Try to imagine your loved one in a dangerous situation. Identify behaviors or words that would give you hope or comfort. Consider whether physical care provided to your loved one is enough to alleviate your fears. Reflect on your past experiences with a family member's illness to determine how the client's husband may feel right now.

8. How does the care of this client compare to other groups of clients with similar problems?

   Identify other clients who have life-threatening conditions, such as cancer, myocardial infarctions, and so forth. Identify clients who may have to deal with the loss of a fetus because of premature birth or other conditions. Discuss commonalities among all people facing possible death or loss of a loved one.

9. What critical thinking skills did you use to answer the questions in this case?

Clarification, reflection, intellectual humility, intellectual empathy, and so on.

Maternal-Newborn Nursing

Vaginal Birth after Cesarean (VBAC)

The client is a 24-year-old woman who is a gravida III, para II and who is at 40 weeks' gestation. She has two healthy children living at home, a 4-year-old and a 3-year-old. Her second pregnancy ended in an emergency cesarean delivery, via an incision through the lower segment of the uterus, due to fetal distress.

The client has no known allergies or chronic health problems. She maintains a well-balanced diet and gained 28 lbs during her pregnancy. She exercises regularly and feels well-prepared to experience labor and a vaginal delivery. As a result, the client's physician has approved her for a VBAC.

Currently, the client has been admitted to the hospital in early labor, with contractions of moderate intensity occurring every 7 to 10 minutes, lasting 45 to 60 seconds. Her husband, a quiet, serious individual, is with her. The nurse assesses the client and reports her findings to the client's physician, who orders an intravenous infusion of dextrose 5% in lactated Ringer's solution.

Vaginal examination of the client reveals that her cervix is 2 cm dilated and 80% effaced. The fetal monitor shows the fetal heart rate varying between 126 to 130 beats per minute (bpm) and has good variability. The client's blood pressure is 130/84, her heart rate is 92 bpm, her respirations are 28 breaths per minute, and her oral temperature is 99.2F.

The client's diagnostic findings are within normal limits.

~~~~

1. What can you infer from the information provided?

   Analyze the subjective and objective data, noting strengths and limitations. Consider the client's physical and emotional status in regard to her pregnancy and delivery. Draw conclusions about the client's readiness for and ability to undergo vaginal delivery of her baby.

2. How can you best enhance the client's comfort and protect her safety?

Review care for a client experiencing a noncomplicated vaginal delivery. Consider assessments that you should make to detect possible complications arising from the client's previous cesarean delivery. Review the Nursing Interventions Classification (NIC) to determine appropriate interventions and nursing activities for the client.

3. How will you know if the client is developing complications?

Review complications occurring from vaginal and postcesarean deliveries. Discuss the need for additional monitoring because of the client's previous cesarean birth, such as monitoring vital signs; performing vaginal examinations; noting appearance of drainage, especially amniotic fluid; evaluating the client's complaints; and noting the development of hemorrhage. Compare normal with abnormal data that may suggest prolonged or nonprogressive labor, a uterine tear, hemorrhage, and so on.

4. How did the physician decide that the client was an appropriate candidate for a VBAC?

Identify contraindications to a VBAC, such as having a previous cesarean with a vertical incision, fetus larger than mother's pelvic dimensions, and so on. Review the 1988 guidelines issued by the American College of Obstetrics and Gynecology (ACOG) for VBAC criteria and aspects that need to be considered. Discuss how the client meets this criteria and describe conditions that must be met during her delivery, such as the presence of a physician who can perform a cesarean within 30 minutes.

5. What fears or concerns may the client and her husband be experiencing about vaginal delivery of their infant?

Discuss the possible positive and negative impact of previous birth experiences on this labor and delivery. Consider the couple's need for a normal birth experience; the amount of support they can provide to one another; and their potential fears regarding the progression of labor, pain associated with labor and delivery, risk of laceration, complications that can occur from VBAC, and the possibility of death of the infant or mother.

6. What critical thinking skills did you use to answer the questions in this case?

Basic support, creativity, intellectual humility, intellectual empathy, and so on.

Nursing Care of Children

Nursing Care of Children
Acute Glomerulonephritis

The client is a normally active 10-year-old boy whose mother is concerned about his recent loss of appetite and complaints of fatigue. Two days ago, he came home from school and slept all evening. Yesterday he didn't want to go to soccer practice, which is most unusual for the client. His temperature this morning was 37.8C orally, so his mother decided to consult her pediatrician.

A physical examination confirmed the client's elevated temperature and revealed a blood pressure of 144/96, a heart rate of 98 beats per minute (bpm), and respirations of 28 breaths per minute. The remainder of the physical examination was unremarkable. Upon questioning the client, his pediatrician learned that the boy had experienced a sore throat about 2 weeks earlier but did not tell his mother for fear of missing his soccer practice and games.

The client's urinalysis is positive for red blood cells and protein. His urine specific gravity is elevated. The client's pediatrician suspects that the client has acute glomerulonephritis and, therefore, prescribes bed rest and daily weights. The pediatrician also obtains a throat culture.

The client's diagnostic findings are as follows:

Urine analysis: urine RBC = 3+; urine protein = 3+; specific gravity = 1.040

~~~~~

1. What are the advantages of collecting more data before making decisions about the client's health status?

   Discuss the need for collecting adequate data prior to making decisions. Examine the possible consequences to the client if treatment is initiated for a problem that does not exist or if the wrong treatment is initiated for a problem that does exist. Consider the need for additional assessments, such as a throat culture, blood chemistry studies, and so on.

2. What is the relationship between the client's previous sore throat and his present symptoms of lethargy, appetite loss, elevated temperature, and elevated blood pressure?

Review the pathophysiology of acute glomerulonephritis, caused by group A β-hemolytic streptococci. Explain how untreated strep throat, from group A β-hemolytic streptococci, can result in the deposit of immune and complement complexes in the kidney basement membrane, causing decreased glomerular filtration and subsequent renal alterations.

3. Why did the client's physician collect a throat culture when the client is no longer complaining of a sore throat?

Discuss the purpose of and information obtained from a throat culture. Consider the need to eradicate the source of the client's glomerulonephritis, which could be a persistent streptococcal infection.

4. Why do you think the client's pediatrician did not prescribe an antibiotic for the client?

Compare kidney inflammation with kidney infection. Describe the need to determine whether the client has a persistent streptococcal throat infection. Discuss antibiotics' lack of effect on inflammatory processes.

5. Why did the pediatrician order daily weights for the client?

Discuss the concept of fluid balance in a 10-year-old child. Identify the best means of determining fluid balance in the child. Compare the measurement of fluid balance in a child with that of an adult.

6. How would you prioritize the information that you need to teach the client's mother?

   Review home care for a child with acute glomerulonephritis. Identify teaching that the client's mother will probably need. Prioritize this teaching using the life-preservation framework or another prioritizing vehicle.

7. Why is it important to perform strep screens on children with sore throat infections?

   Describe the purpose of a strep screen. Explain why the strep screen is a reliable choice for diagnosing a streptococcal throat infection, considering clinical manifestations of such infections are not specific to strep throat. Discuss the advantages of treating a streptococcal infection immediately, such as preventing complications including acute glomerulonephritis.

8. If you were the client's mother, how might you feel about your child's illness?

   Consider how you might feel if the client was your child, for example, guilty over not recognizing the child's sore throat and, subsequently, delaying medical care. Discuss interventions to decrease the mother's feelings of guilt or inadequacy.

9. What attitude and cognitive critical thinking skills did you use to address this case?

   Faith in reason, intellectual empathy, reasoning, clarification, and so on.

Nursing Care of Children
Bronchopulmonary Dysplasia (BPD) in Premature Infant

The client is an 11-month-old girl, delivered at 24 weeks' gestation by Cesarean section. Her premature birth was necessitated by fetal distress related to spontaneous rupture of the mother's fetal membranes a month prior to the client's birth. The baby weighed 2 kg upon delivery. Shortly after her birth, she was intubated with an endotracheal tube and transferred to the neonatal intensive care unit (NICU). At the age of 2 weeks, the client underwent a second intubation following an unsuccessful attempt to wean her from the endotracheal tube to a nasal cannula. The client's respiratory status did not improve; consequently, she received a tracheostomy and became ventilator dependent. With prolonged exposure to high-pressure oxygenation, the client developed BPD.

Currently, the client maintains a fair status in her dependency on the ventilator. She weighs 9.2 kg. Her oxygen is set at 38%, with a positive end-expiratory pressure (PEEP) of 22 and pressure limits of 50. Throughout the day she requires suctioning, which produces thick, pale, yellow mucus. She is being fed by a gastrostomy tube due to severe gastroesophageal reflux (GER). The NICU nurse feeds her 240 mL of Neocare, a 24-calorie formula, over a 2-hour period every 4 hours. The client receives nothing by mouth. She has no known allergies, and her immunizations are up-to-date. In the past 11 months, she has received antibiotic therapy for *Streptococcus a.* infections. Her medications include 2 puffs of albuterol every 4 hours, 1 puff of cromolyn and Atrovent every 8 hours, an iron supplement daily, 140 mg of Diuril every 12 hours, and 14 mg of Aldactone every 12 hours. A child-life therapist interacts with the client daily to work on her social, cognitive, and motor skills.

The client's mother is not married and has two other children, ages 7 and 3. They all live with the children's maternal grandmother in her five-room house. The client's mother usually visits her daughter once a day and insists on performing her morning care. The baby has personal floral bed linens, a flowered dress, and neatly brushed hair without accessories. After providing this personal care, the mother and siblings sit, talk, and stroke the client's face.

Upon examination, the client reveals coarse, regular, and unlabored respirations. Her oxygen saturation remains between 96% and 100% except during suctioning. Her capillary refill time is 2 seconds. Bowel sounds are present in all four quadrants. Her urine is pale yellow, and her bowel movements are regular. Her tracheostomy and gastrostomy sites are both clean and dry. The client reacts to her mother's voice and occasionally responds to her siblings and other people. She smiles appropriately and makes eye contact with care providers and others. The baby is able to grasp objects and play with toys suspended from a string above the crib. She can roll onto her side and displays no head lag when she is carried. However, the client is unable to sit unless supported and is incapable of speaking or following simple commands. In addition, she is unable to transport herself or crawl, and she does not display a palmer grasp.

The client's diagnostic findings are as follows:

Respiratory status: stable via ventilator assist

Chronic BPD is a destabilizing factor in respiratory function.

~~~~

1. Could the client's BPD have been prevented?

   Review the etiologic factors and pathophysiology of BPD. Examine the relationship between exposure to high-pressure oxygen and the development of BPD. Consider the iatrogenic nature of BPD. Discuss methods to support premature infants without the use of high-pressure oxygen.

2. How are the client's BPD and GER related?

   Review the pathophysiology of BPD and its complications. Discuss the impact of BPD on the developing neonate. Identify the impact of one condition on the other.

3. Considering the client's compromised respiratory status, what precautions should you take when suctioning her?

   - Review the procedure for suctioning an infant. Consider the need for absolute asepsis, hyperoxygenation prior to suctioning, use of a 4-cm suction catheter, suctioning no longer than 5 seconds, and so on.

   - Discuss the client's susceptibility to infection and the impact of any infection on her respiratory status.

4. What important conditions should you monitor to ensure they fall within appropriate parameters and thus avoid further compromising the client's health?

   Review assessment parameters for all body systems in an infant. Consider monitoring intake and output levels, length and weight, serum electrolytes, skin integrity, stoma appearances, and developmental patterns. Note possible sources of infection, sensory or other deprivations, further respiratory compromise, and so on.

5. How does the client's physical and social development compare to other infants her age?

   Review the normal growth and development patterns for 11-month-old infants. Compare those findings with the client's data. Note any deficits in her development, such as her inability to sit or crawl, to follow simple commands, and so on.

6. How is the client's lack of palmer grasp significant?

   Define "palmer grasp." Review the significance of the palmer grasp and the age at which infants generally develop this ability. Discuss the consequences of not developing a palmer grasp, such as lack of involvement in sequential play or inability to manipulate objects or remove them from tight-fitting enclosures.

7. Why did the physician prescribe Diuril and Aldactone for this client?

   Investigate the actions and common uses for the medications Aldactone and Diuril. Relate your findings to the client's situation.

8. Would an interdisciplinary team conference benefit the client and her mother?

   Identify individuals who are generally involved in interdisciplinary team conferences, such as the client's nurse, physical therapist, child-life therapist, physician, social worker, and so on. Examine the benefit of each of these individuals in planning care for the client and providing assistance to her mother. Consider how you might feel in this situation if you were the mother or the nurse. Determine the value of such a conference to this child and her family.

9. What effect may the client's health and social condition have on the parent-infant and infant-sibling relationships?

   Identify the strengths and limitations of the client's relationship with her mother and siblings. Discuss how infant bonding and relationship development generally progress for the normal infant and compare this process with the client's relationships and their development. Identify factors that are inhibiting the client's interactions. Create ways to enhance her interactions.

10. What attitude and cognitive critical thinking skills did you use to address the problems in this case?

    Divergent thinking, reflection, intellectual courage, intellectual sense of justice, and so on.

Nursing Care of Children
Cultural Differences and Breastfeeding

The client is the 22-year-old mother of a newborn baby boy. Her son was 2.5 kg at birth and is being seen at the well baby clinic for his 4-week appointment. The client immigrated to the United States from Bangladesh 2 years ago. She attended prenatal classes and followed routine protocols to prepare for a vaginal delivery, however, a cesarean section was necessary. The client was disappointed but agreed that she felt safe with the physician's decision. The client decided in prenatal classes to breastfeed her baby and is doing so successfully. Her mother-in-law is visiting from Bangladesh and has been here since the baby's birth.

While visiting with the nurse practitioner, the client confesses her anxiety about breastfeeding her baby. She states that her mother-in-law disapproves of breastfeeding and frequently complains that the baby is not receiving adequate nourishment. She describes the baby's discomfort after feedings, which she believes are stomach cramps. She states that now she is worried that the baby is not receiving adequate amounts of milk. In addition, the client is receiving no support from her husband, who agrees with his mother.

~~~~

1. What conclusions can you draw about the client and her situation?

   Consider possibilities, such as: the client being prevented from making her own decisions, the client's mother-in-law and husband being uninformed, or cultural differences influencing their comments.

2. What data support your conclusions?

Review your conclusions and identify data that formed the basis of your conclusions. Decide if you have adequate data to draw conclusions. Discuss the
need to collect adequate data prior to drawing any conclusions.

3. What is the possible relationship between baby's discomfort after feedings
and his intake of milk?

Review the benefits and possible complications associated with breastfeeding,
including the impact of the mother's anxiety and diet on the breast-fed
infant, the possibility of a milk allergy, and so on. Review the problem of
colic and factors that contribute to its development.

4. What are the advantages and disadvantages of breastfeeding compared to
bottle-feeding?

Investigate the nutritional, immunologic, and emotional benefits associated
with breastfeeding versus bottle-feeding with formula. Discuss the manner in
which various cultures view the process of breastfeeding. Identify cultures
that support breastfeeding and those that oppose it. Discuss disadvantages of
breastfeeding, such as the mother's anxiety, need for privacy, adequacy of the
amount of milk, and so on.

5. Discuss whether you could effectively intervene to support the client's desire to breastfeed her infant if milk allergy is not an issue.

   Evaluate whether further education would impact the mother-in-law's or son's view of breastfeeding. Discuss the need to support this family's cultural beliefs and the need for nurses, in general, to support cultural differences. Consider the impact of defending a client when such an act may negate cultural beliefs. Decide what impact you could have in this situation.

6. What affective and cognitive critical thinking skills did you use to address this case?

   Faith in reason, clarification, basic support, divergent thinking, and so on.

Nursing Care of Children
Gastroesophageal Reflux (GER)

The client is a 10-month-old baby boy who has GER and chronic lung disease related to premature birth. He is receiving oxygen through a nasal cannula at 2 liters per minute. His oxygen saturation ranges from 95% to 100%. His respiratory rate is within normal limits for his age. Due to his GER, the client has recently undergone placement of a gastro-jejunostomy tube. He is able to receive formula, which is provided at the rate of 30 mL per hour over a 4-hour time period three times each day. Presently, the client is being considered for discharge to his parents, who visit him daily. The client has two older siblings at home.

~~~~

1. Why is it important to maintain strict intake and output on the client?

   Discuss the importance of maintaining an infant's fluid balance and the problems associated with inadequate fluid balance. Consider the length of time it takes for an infant to develop fluid imbalance, hypovolemia, or cellular dehydration. Review the importance of monitoring urinary output and insensible losses to determine fluid replacement needs.

2. What conditions and related parameters should you monitor to evaluate the adequacy of the client's feedings?

   Identify assessments and related parameters that enable you to evaluate the adequacy of breastfeeding, bottle-feeding, and alternative methods of feeding for infants. Consider the infant's weight gain or loss, ability to tolerate feedings, ability to increase feedings with growth, appearance and consistency of stools, fussiness, and so on.

3. How will the nurse know when the client's mother is ready to care for her child independently?

Review verbal and nonverbal signs of interest in learning, interest in performing self-care, or interest in performing care for another person. Identify signs that indicate the mother's interest in her infant, her interest in assisting with her infant's care, her questions or search for printed materials, her ability to change her infant's dressing or assist with his tube feedings, her verbalizations of eagerness to take her infant home, and so on.

4. What should the nurse teach the client's mother about signs and symptoms that indicate she should contact the client's pediatrician?

* Review the pathophysiolgy and common complications associated with tube feedings and the presence of a gastrostomy jejunostomy tube.

* Decide which problems need to be reported.

* Design a teaching method to convey such information to the mother. Consider including information regarding normal care and findings, signs and symptoms of complications, access to routine or emergency care, and so on.

5. What attitude and cognitive critical thinking skills did you use to address the client's case?

Divergent thinking, creativity, reasoning, and intellectual empathy.

Nursing Care of Children
Heroin and Cocaine Addiction

The client is a 5-month-old baby girl who was born prematurely at 31 weeks and has been admitted to a pediatric hospital with the medical diagnosis of bradycardia, risk for sudden infant death syndrome (SIDS), and gastroesophageal reflux (GER). She was exposed to cocaine and heroin in utero.

On admission, the client was below average for her weight; however, she has been gaining approximately 100 g per day. She receives formula containing 28 calories per ounce through a nasogastric tube at 110 mL per hour every 3 hours. A cardiac-respiratory monitor is attached to the client at all times, and a pulse oximeter is constantly in use. Bradycardiac alarms are set at 80 beats per minute (bpm), and her crib side rails are up.

The client is in the custody of her grandmother who visits infrequently. Therefore, professional and volunteer care providers are her primary source of interaction. Child-life specialists visit the client daily to develop her social, cognitive, and motor skills. Quiet time for rest is allotted each day. A major portion of the client's time is spent in a crib. While awake, and usually in a prone position, she plays with toys attached to a string within reach. Other social activities involve rattles, music, and pictures of faces in the playroom.

Upon examination, the client reveals oxygen saturation levels consistently above 98%, and she has no signs of respiratory distress. Her capillary refill time is less than 2 seconds, her blood pressure is 90/52, and her pulse is strong and ranges between 110 and 140 bpm. Her urine output is normal, with wet diapers every 2 to 3 hours. Her urine specific gravity is 1.021. In addition, her bowel sounds are present, and she has no abdominal distention. The client has one to two stools each day, most of which are loose but test negative for occult blood.

The client's diagnostic findings are as follows:

Neurological status: within normal limits

Respiratory status: no significant distress

Gastrointestinal status: no significant distress

~~~~

1. What is the primary cause of the client's current state of health?

   Analyze all data about the client and separate the information into physical and social categories. Review the common problems associated with premature births. Compare and contrast the client's data with expectations for a premature infant. Draw conclusions about the problems that the client is experiencing that are specifically related to her prematurity or to her exposure to cocaine and heroin in utero.

2. Why it is necessary to feed the client through a gastrostomy jejunostomy tube since she is awake and responsive to external stimuli?

   Review the pathophysiology and treatment of GER. Discuss complications that may occur from oral feeding and the need for maintaining adequate nutrition in a 5-month-old baby.

3. On the basis of the data supplied, what is the client's current stage of development?

   Review data related to the client's developmental stage. Review Erikson's or another theorist's stages of childhood development. Compare the client's developmental traits with those considered normal for a 5-month-old infant. Identify traits that are consistent and inconsistent with normal development.

4. What is the relationship between the client's bradycardia, her prematurity, and her increased risk for SIDS?

Review known risk factors for SIDS. Compare those factors with characteristics that predispose the client to the development of SIDS. Note the impact of immure cardiac and respiratory systems on infants with other problems, such as drug exposure.

5. What precautions will the client's grandmother need to take in regard to her risk for SIDS when she takes the client home from the hospital?

Review care of the infant at risk for developing SIDS. Discuss precautions that can reduce the possibility of SIDS for all infants, including babies with no known risk factors. Consider position of the infant for sleep, using monitoring equipment, and so on.

6. Considering the client's family structure, what social needs do you think she will have when she is discharged from the hospital?

Review the typical social needs of a 5-month-old infant. Draw possible conclusions about the degree of physical care, sensory stimulation, and affection that she received prior to this hospitalization and whether her needs were being met. Consider the impact of the grandmother's other responsibilities and the absence of parents on the client's social needs.

7. What outcomes might you predict regarding the client's future?

Review the data related to the client's support systems. Consider the magnitude of the client's physical problems, the absence of her mother, the infrequent visits from her grandmother, the possible lack of bonding, the financial burden the client will place on her grandmother, and so on. Speculate about the probability of the client becoming a ward of the state. Weigh the advantages and disadvantages of placing the client in foster care with the future possibility of adoption.

8. What attitude or cognitive critical thinking skills did you use to address the questions in this case?

   Intellectual sense of justice, intellectual courage, reasoning, divergent thinking, clarification, and so on.

The client is a 3-year-old boy who presented to the emergency department with fever, abdominal distention, poor feeding, and general gastrointestinal symptoms. The client's birth history revealed complications of preeclampsia, induced labor, and subsequent cesarean birth. Hirschsprung's disease was revealed about 48 hours after his birth when he failed to pass meconium stool. One week later, his physician performed a temporary ileostomy by using a Soave's pull-through surgical procedure. Currently, the client has been admitted to a children's hospital with the diagnosis of enterocolitis secondary to Hirschsprung's disease.

The client is fed 90 mL of Isocal, containing 28 calories per ounce, every 3 hours by mouth. His physician recently advanced his feeding from 26 calories per ounce given both orally and by gavage. The oral feedings have not resulted in aspiration or respiratory distress; however, the change to oral feedings has been slow and requires frequent burping.

Child-life activities for the client are limited to once a day, during which time he practices grasping a rattle, batting a mobile, and maximizing full range-of-motion activities. In the afternoons, he observes quiet time and generally sleeps. He is active for a short period following his rest time.

The client's father works full-time at a job that provides health insurance, and he habitually smokes cigarettes. The client's mother works part-time at a nearby grocery store. Neither parent finished high school. The client is their first and only child. Due to lack of transportation, the client's parents visit infrequently. They continue to be unsure and inexperienced with caring for an ostomy or a chronically ill child but state they are trying to adjust to his care. They have applied for public aid to help with expenses.

Upon examination, the client reveals oxygenation perfusion within normal limits and a regular respiratory rate at 38 breaths per minute. His nares are patent, and his breathing is nonlabored. The client's apical rate is 140 beats per minute (bpm) without murmurs. His skin is dry and pink. Bowel sounds are present in all quadrants, and his ileostomy drains approximately 100 mL of loose, brown, seedy stool each shift. There is no indication of diarrhea or constipation. The client's abdominal girth measurement is negative for distention. He voids two to three times per shift, and his 12-hour urine specific gravities are normal.

The client's diagnostic findings are as follows:

Cardiovascular status: within normal limits

Gastrointestinal status: no significant distress

The client is ready to be discharged and go home.

~~~~

1. What nursing concerns would you have about this child even if you did not know his medical diagnosis?

   Cluster the data into related categories and develop a problem list. Decide which problems are related to the client's medical diagnosis and which ones are related to oral feedings, parental interactions, his ostomy, and so on. List those problems that could be addressed without knowing his medical diagnosis, such as fluid balance, skin care around his stoma, maintenance of ideal body weight for his age, and parental ability to care for his needs.

2. How does the client's gastrointestinal tract differ from that of a normal child?

   Review the pathophysiology of Hirschsprung's disease. Discuss alterations that occur in the colon of infants affected by the disease. Identify clinical manifestations commonly associated with Hirschsprung's disease. Compare the textbook picture of the disease with the clinical manifestations experienced by the client.

3. When should you change the client's ostomy bag?

   Review care of an ostomy, including care of the skin around it and use of ostomy appliances. Identify recommendations for changing the ostomy appliance, such as every shift, every day, or every time the contents leak, the bag is full, or odor or gas is present.

4. What data suggest that the client is within, or not within, the appropriate developmental stage for his age?

   Review Ericson's or another theorist's stages of childhood development. Analyze data that specifically address the client's developmental level. Compare the client's development with parameters for the normal 3-year-old child. Identify characteristics that are consistent with normal development and areas where the client may be behind other 3-year-olds.

5. How are Hirschsprung's disease and enterocolitis related?

   Define the term "enterocolitis." Investigate the common causes of enterocolitis. Review the complications commonly associated with Hirschsprung's disease. Consider factors in the client's environment that, when coupled with his disease, may have increased his risk for developing enterocolitis.

6. Which assessments for the client should take priority to prevent further problems or complications?

   Review the problems and complications commonly associated with an ileostomy and enterocolitis in a child. Identify pertinent assessments and monitoring parameters. Consider the client's skin integrity, developmental abilities, intake and output levels, fluid and electrolytes, nutrition, parental interactions, and so on.

7. What impact does the father's smoking have on the client's current condition and overall health status?

Discuss the impact of secondhand smoke on the child's respiratory status. Identify possible complications that the client could develop related to his father's tobacco use using your knowledge of pediatrics, immunology, and chronic illness.

8. What government programs could benefit the client and his parents?

Investigate community and governmental services available in your area, including public health, child welfare, and social and rehabilitative services. Explore the feasibility of referring the client's parents to these agencies. Identify specific types of assistance each agency may offer.

9. How might your own biases regarding the client and his situation impact your ability to work with his parents or care for the child?

Identify your opinions or beliefs about the client's parents and their ability to adequately provide for the client's needs. Consider both their strengths and limitations. Explore your feelings about the client's father smoking around the client, their inability to visit, and so on. Discuss how both negative and positive biases can impact your care of the child and parents.

10. What attitude and cognitive critical thinking skills did you use to address this case?

Divergent thinking, reasoning, clarification, and intellectual humility.

Nursing Care of Children
Immunizations

The client is a 2-year-old female toddler who has been in good health since birth. The client's mother works part-time; therefore, the client stays next door with the neighbor twice weekly. The client enjoys being at the neighbor's house because her 3-year-old friend lives there.

The client's mother is conscientious about her daughter's health, making sure that the client stays home when she is not feeling well, eats a well-balanced diet, gets adequate sleep, and receives her immunizations on time. Thus far, the client has received the hepatitis B, diphtheria-tetanus-pertussis (DTP), *Haemophilus influenzae b* (Hib), mumps-measles-rubella (MMR), and oral poliovirus (OPV) vaccines. The client's mother recognizes that her daughter will need further immunizations prior to starting kindergarten.

During a recent conversation with her neighbor, the client's mother learned that her neighbor's daughter has not received any of her childhood immunizations. The neighbors fear that the foreign substances contained in vaccines will be more harmful to their daughter than the childhood diseases. As support for her belief, the neighbor explained that her daughter had measles last year and recovered without incidence.

~~~~~

1. How are the two children's immunity to measles similar or different?

   Investigate the differences between actively acquired artificial immunity and actively acquired natural immunity. Identify which child has which type of immunity. Explain how contracting a disease and receiving an immunization results in the same type of immunity, but with different durations. Explain why the child receiving the vaccine needed more than one immunization.

2. If these children lived in your state, what immunizations would be required before they start kindergarten?

Call your local health department and investigate immunization requirements for your county and state. Using the Internet, investigate the recommendations of the Centers for Disease Control and Prevention (CDC) for childhood immunizations.

3. If you were the client's mother, what information could you offer to your neighbor about the risks and benefits of immunization?

Investigate the actions and side effects of several vaccines, such as the MMR or OPV vaccines. List and compare the potential harmful effects and benefits of such vaccines. Decide which information would be most useful in convincing the neighbor to immunize her child.

4. What actions should you take prior to giving any child or adult an immunization?

Investigate nursing care for the child or adult receiving immunizations. Consider the presence of infections or fever, contraindications, scheduling, permission from the parent, and so on.

5. When should parents contact the primary caregiver or pediatrician following their child's immunization?

Review the possible complications associated with vaccines. Consider both systemic and local reactions. List clinical manifestations that you should report to the physician.

6. How do adult and older-adult immunization schedules differ from childhood immunization schedules?

   Obtain immunization schedules for adults and older adults from your local public health department. Compare the recommended immunizations with those of children.

7. Do you think that the neighbor should be persuaded to have her child immunized?

   State your opinion. Consider whether your opinion reflects your own personal biases. Offer facts that support your opinion.

8. What attitude and cognitive critical thinking skills did you use to address this case?

   Clarification, divergent thinking, basic support, and intellectual humility.

Nursing Care of Children
Iron Deficiency Anemia

The client is an 8-month-old baby girl, admitted to a community hospital pediatric unit to rule out iron deficiency anemia. She lives in a single-parent home with her mother, grandmother, and two older siblings. Anemia is suspected because of the client's fatigue during feedings and play and her pale skin. Her weight is appropriate for her age at 50% on the growth chart issued by the National Center for Health Statistics (NCHS). The client has started solid foods recently, and has been given cow's milk since 1 month of age.

The client's diagnostic findings are as follows:

Chemistry profile: TIBC 450 μg/dL, serum Fe 12 μg/dL.

Hematology: Hgb 8 g/dL, 30%.

Her admission orders call for oral ferrous sulfate, vitamin C supplements, oxygen by nasal cannula, and iron-fortified formula and cereals.

~~~~

1. How can the client's weight be appropriate for her age with a condition such as iron deficiency anemia?

   Explore factors leading to iron deficiency anemia in infants. Speculate about the possible iron sources or lack thereof in the client's diet. Identify nutrients that may cause normal weight gain but will not provide adequate iron intake. Discuss the possibility that the client has an iron malabsorption problem.

2. How are the client's clinical manifestations and iron deficiency anemia related?

   Review the need for iron in the human body, including the production of red blood cells (RBCs). Discuss the relationship between adequate RBC production, hemoglobin, and oxygen-carrying capacity of the blood. Identify common clinical manifestations associated with reduced hemoglobin and hematocrit, such as fatigue.

3. How are the client's laboratory findings significant?

   Review each of the laboratory tests ordered for the client, noting normal and abnormal values. Compare normal values with the client's values, identifying abnormal results. Relate each abnormal finding with the client's symptoms.

4. Why is the client receiving oxygen?

   * Explore the relationship between RBCs and oxygen-carrying capacity. Consider the need to increase the number of RBCs or increase the oxygen supply to the existing RBCs to rectify the client's condition.

   * Review the effect of oxygenation on energy levels.

5. What teaching or other care is necessary for the client's mother?

   Consider the possibility of knowledge deficits regarding the client's diet, such as her use of cow's milk. Consider that the mother may feel guilty about her care of the client and will require a nonjudgmental attitude from you. Think about whether the client's siblings are also at risk for nutritional deficiencies and explore ways of obtaining such information.

6. What are the advantages of delaying judgment about the mother's care of this child until all the facts are available?

Discuss the reasons to refrain from making judgments about the mother's parenting abilities until further data is available, including the dangers inherent in forming premature conclusions. Consider the benefits of having enough data to draw accurate conclusions.

7. What affective and cognitive critical thinking skills did you use for this case?

Faith in reason, basic support, clarification, and reasoning.

Nursing Care of Children
Otitis Media

The client is an 11-month-old infant who resides with her mother, father, and three siblings. The client and her 2-year-old sister attend day care because both of their parents work. Her other siblings are school-aged and attend the same day care after school. The client's mother breast-fed her for the first 2 months of her life but weaned her to a bottle when she started back to work.

Last month, the client developed an upper respiratory infection after being exposed to another infected child at the day care. Several days later her mother took her to her pediatrician for fussiness, crying, pulling on her right ear, and fever. Upon examination, the nurse practitioner noted a red, bulging tympanic membrane with a small amount of purulent drainage from the client's right ear. She prescribed oral ampicillin to be given for 10 days.

Today the nurse practitioner is seeing the client again for similar symptoms. Two days ago, the baby became fussy and began pulling at her ear. Yesterday she refused to eat well. This morning, the client had a fever that prompted her mother to return for further care. The client's history reveals that her father is a moderate to heavy smoker.

~~~~

1. What risk factors does the client have for acute otitis media?

   Review factors that predispose children to develop otitis media. Review the client's data and make a list of her risk factors, considering her exposure to other children, her bottle feedings, and her father's smoking.

2. How does passive cigarette smoke increase the client's risk for ear infections?

Research the effects of cigarette smoke on the respiratory tract and subsequent ear infections in children. Consider impaired mucociliary function, congestion of soft nasopharyngeal tissues, and so on.

3. How does acute otitis media differ from chronic otitis media?

Review the four types of otitis media. Consider the onset, frequency, duration, and clinical manifestations of each type. Discuss criteria that differentiate each type of otitis media.

4. How are upper respiratory infections and otitis media related?

Review the pathophysiology of respiratory infections and otitis media. Consider how an upper respiratory infection often precedes the development of otitis media. Describe how infection leads to edema of the mucous membranes in the eustachian tube, which provides a medium for further infection.

5. What priority nursing diagnoses apply to the child with otitis media?

On the basis of your of pathophysiology review of otitis media, list actual and potential nursing diagnoses. Using a suitable framework, prioritize the nursing diagnoses.

6. How could you approach the client's father about his cigarette smoking and the dangers it poses to his child?

Reflect on any of your past experiences in which you had to change a habit. Identify strategies that helped you change and those that made you resistant to change. Consider the ease with which habits are changed. Discuss the need for parents to recognize that their habits may be harmful to their children. Identify various approaches for bringing the father's smoking to his attention without being judgemental.

7. What attitude and cognitive critical thinking skills did you use to address this case?

Basic support, reflection, reasoning, and intellectual empathy.

Nursing Care of Children
Pneumonia and Asthma

The client is a 15-year-old female high-school student who was admitted to the hospital with complaints of shortness of breath and right-sided chest pain upon breathing. She states that she has had influenza for 3 days. She has had a history of asthma since the age of 6, and admits that she smokes a half pack of cigarettes per day. Her parents each smoke a pack a day.

She is currently receiving intravenous (IV) fluids, 800 mg of IV vancomycin every 12 hours, 10 incentive spirometer treatments per hour while awake, and chest physiotherapy. She is not on oxygen therapy. Her heart rate is 80 beats per minute (bpm), her respiratory rate is 24 breaths per minute, and her blood pressure is 110/70. Her skin is pale but warm, and her capillary refill time is 2 seconds with no clubbing. She is urinating approximately 400 mL of clear yellow urine per shift, and she is maintaining a normal bowel movement pattern.

Her diagnostic findings are as follows:

Hematology: RBC 3.56, WBC 11.8, Hgb 11.2 g/dL, and Hct 32.7%

The client complains of fatigue and muscle weakness. Her cough produces white, thick sputum, and her sputum culture on admission confirms the diagnosis of streptococcal pneumonia. Plans are being made to discharge the client to her home in 3 days.

~~~~

1. Of the data provided, what important information is missing?

   Cluster the data into related categories and develop a problem list. Identify further data that are needed to confirm your conclusions about the client's health problems. Consider additional data such as lung sounds, fever, chills, and so on.

2. How is streptococcal pneumonia similar to and different from other types of pneumonia?

Review the etiology and pathophysiology of pneumonia. Compare the clinical manifestations and laboratory data found with bacterial pneumonia to viral pneumonia. How does an intact immune system affect a person's susceptibility to infectious agents that can cause pneumonia?

3. What factors place the client at increased risk for continued respiratory problems?

Review the etiology of childhood asthma and contributing factors that lead to its development. Discuss the impact of firsthand and secondhand smoke on the lungs of a child and an asthmatic.

4. How do you feel about parents who place their children at risk for health problems?

Examine your own feelings about parents smoking around their children and allowing their children to smoke. Consider whether your feelings toward the parents change if the child has asthma. Decide if your reaction represents a positive or negative bias. Identify other lifestyle habits that can place children at risk for health problems.

5. How can you best approach the client and her parents about her risk factors?

Discuss various methods of approaching both the client and her parents about cigarette smoking, such as direct discussion, booklets or other written materials, and so on. Discuss the need to remain factual and nonjudgmental. Explore how your attitude can influence the manner in which you relate to clients' parents who place their children at risk for disease.

6. What attitude and cognitive critical thinking skills did you use to address this case?

Divergent thinking, clarification, basic support, and intellectual humility.

Nursing Care of Children
Respiratory Distress Syndrome

The client is a 7-week-old baby boy admitted to the pediatric unit from the nursery for severe respiratory distress that developed after an emergency delivery caused by fetal distress. The client's mother relates a history of treatment for oral candidiasis infection (thrush) early in her pregnancy and vaginal bleeding at 30 weeks' gestation, which resulted in an emergency cesarean delivery. The client weighed 1.69 kg and had an Apgar of 6 at 1 minute and 8 at 5 minutes. In obvious respiratory distress, the baby was intubated and admitted to the neonatal intensive care unit (NICU). There, the client experienced several episodes of apnea, which were resolved with oral theophylline. The medication was discontinued after 1 week.

Currently, the client is attached to cardiac-respiratory monitors and a pulse oximeter. His mother breastfeeds him every 3 to 4 hours. The parents have been instructed that if the client requires feeding supplements at home, they should give him formula, containing 20 calories per ounce, using a bottle with regular full-term nipples. The physician is considering the need for a nasogastric tube if the client loses weight. The client's medications include ampicillin and cefotaxime.

Since the father works two jobs, his mother stays with the baby. She understands and speaks little English. The client's room is adorned with pictures of the Virgin Mary, lit and unlit candles, a rosary, Bible, and several religious pictures. A translator is occasionally needed when new procedures are being discussed with the client's mother.

Upon examination, the client's respirations are 40 breaths per minute, which are generally coarse with subcostal and intercostal retractions. His oxygen saturations range from 96% to 100%. His body temperature is 96F rectally, his heart rate is 154 beats per minute (bpm), and his blood pressure is 38/16. His radial pulse in his left arm is faint, and his hand is cyanotic.

The client's diagnostic findings are as follows:

Blood cultures: Negative for pathogens

Urine cultures: Negative for pathogens

Capillary blood gas: pH 7.38, $PaCO_2$ 29 mm Hg, PaO_2 40 mm Hg

~~~~

1. How are the client's respiratory distress and premature delivery related?

   Review the normal development of the embryo and note those systems that are not fully mature until 36 weeks' gestation. Identify aspects of the client's respiratory system that need further development, such as surfactant. Consider the concept of alveolar compliance.

2. What is the significance of a 1-minute Apgar score of 6?

   Discuss the importance of Apgar scoring and conditions that must be met for each point on the scale. While considering the impact of a premature birth, draw conclusions about the client's Apgar score of 6. Discuss other conditions that can result in lowered Apgar scores. Consider factors that improved the client's score within 5 minutes of birth.

3. How does the client differ from the normal newborn infant of his age?

   Review assessment findings for the normal newborn infant. Compare the findings for a normal newborn with those of a premature infant. Discuss both physical and psychosocial deficits that may exist in a 7-week-old premature infant that will not be found in the normal newborn.

4. What priority problems must you anticipate and how will you detect such problems?

   Analyze the client's assessment findings, laboratory data, and history. Identify risks to his health, such as his exposure to Candida, the aggressive use of antibiotic therapy, his compromised respiratory status, and so on. Consider potential physical and psychosocial problems, such as increased risk for infection, sudden infant death syndrome (SIDS), or nutritional deficits, delayed bonding related to prolonged hospitalization, and inadequate sensory stimulation. Describe the mother's needs, such as her need to understand and communicate.

5. Why is the client's physician considering a nasogastric tube for the client when he is nursing and able to ingest milk?

   Calculate the number of calories and amount of fats, carbohydrates, and proteins essential for growth of a preterm infant. Compare those requirements with the amount of milk the client is receiving from his mother and his supplements. Consider nutritional deficits that may be occurring, the degree that the client is capable of sucking and ingesting adequate amounts of milk, and his increased caloric needs in his present state, etc.

6. If the client was your baby and you were unable to communicate with his caregivers, how might you feel?

   Reflect on past experiences in which you did not understand directions or the terminology. Think about the feelings that were most apparent to you. Consider emotions you experienced during those circumstances, such as frustration, anxiety, fear, mistrust, and anger. Speculate about how the client's mother is feeling and relate those potential feelings to her religious expressions.

7. How might you support the client's mother considering she may not be able to fully understand words of encouragement?

Explore the effects of cultural diversity on nursing practice and nurse-patient interactions. Identify gestures that are universally known and nonverbal language that can convey caring and support, such as touch, smiling, and nods. Identify sentiments that can be conveyed nonverbally versus those that require the use of an interpreter.

8. What attitude and cognitive critical thinking skills did you use to address the client's case?

Intellectual empathy, intellectual courage, divergent thinking, reasoning, basic support, reflection, and so on.

Nursing Care of Children
Septic Osteomyelitis

The client is a 6-year-old boy who was admitted to the hospital for right knee osteoseptic arthritis, placement of a Hickman catheter, and diagnostic arthroscopy with possible drainage. The client's condition first presented as osteomyelitis at the age of 1. Since then, he has been riding his tricycle, running, and playing catch. He attends school and participates in field trips. He remains mobile in the hospital with the temporary use of a wheelchair. His activities also include physical, child-life, and occupational therapy on a daily basis. He performs most of his own care.

The client is stable with an apical rate of 82 beats per minute (bpm), respirations of 20 breaths per minute, and an oral temperature of 96.8F. His only medication is intravenous cefazolin. His diet is supplemented with multivitamins and iron. Every day, his nurse changes his sterile dressings over his Hickman insertion site. His bowel functions are regular, and intake and output monitoring is not necessary. The client eats a variety of foods; however, he has a large amount of candy that he consumes at will.

~~~~

1. How is septic osteomyelitis different from other forms of arthritis, such as juvenile or rheumatoid arthritis?

   Review the etiology, pathophysiology, and clinical manifestations associated with several types of arthritis that can affect children. Note similarities and differences between these types of arthritis. Compare the incidence of developing septic osteomyelitis with other forms and compare and contrast their collaborative management. Discuss the common causes of septic arthritis, such as infection by Hemophilus influenzae, staphylococcus, and Escherichia coli.

2. What are the benefits of performing diagnostic arthroscopy?

   Review the purpose of a diagnostic arthroscopy. Discuss the need to identify the causative agent involved in septic arthritis to provide the most appropriate antimicrobial therapy.

3. Why is it necessary to hospitalize the client considering intravenous antibiotics can be safely administered at home?

   * Consider the spectrum of care that must be provided prior to initiating home-administered intravenous antibiotics.

   * Review the procedure for insertion of a Hickman catheter and precautions necessary for its care.

   * Consider the need for teaching the client and his mother about care of the catheter, symptoms of infection, administration of medications, and other important details before home care can be considered.

4. Does the client's intake of candy have any influence on the outcome of his care?

   Explore the relationship between nutrition, healing, and the immune response. Discuss the need for maintaining the correct ratio of nutrients to facilitate growth and healing. Describe the negative impact of a diet consisting primarily of candy, such as dental caries, hyperactivity, and so on.

5. What attitude and cognitive critical thinking skills did you use to address this case?

   Clarification, basic support, reasoning, and so on.

Nursing Care of Children
Surgical Preparation

The client is an 8-year-old child who was admitted this morning for a tonsillectomy and adenoidectomy. His pediatrician and parents made the decision to remove his tonsils and adenoids following 2 years of repeated sore throats, tonsillar hypertrophy, and enlarged adenoids, which resulted in difficulty swallowing and breathing. He has no allergies and is in good health otherwise.

Last evening, the client joined four other children for a "surgery party" to tour the operating and recovery rooms and ask questions. The client is aware that he will have a sore throat when he awakens and will have an ice collar in place. He says he is a little afraid but is looking forward to eating ice cream this evening.

His parents have given informed consent for his surgery, and the client has also assented to the surgery. His vital signs are stable and within normal parameters for a child his age. He has urinated and is ready to be transported to the surgical suite.

~~~~

1. How does the client's assent for surgery differ from his parents informed consent?

   Define the term "assent." Investigate the meaning of "informed consent." Consider that assent is usually verbal agreement given by minor children, whereas informed consent is given by parents or guardians. Discuss the concept of assent as an ethical requirement designed to protect the rights of children.

2. Why is it important to include children in the surgical consent process?

Discuss the benefits derived from informing children of procedures or surgery, such as eliciting cooperation with preparations, nurturing feelings of respect and importance, and so on. Discuss the risks involved in not including children in the decision-making process, such as increasing the child's fear, anxiety, and so forth.

3. How does preoperative preparation of a child differ from that of an adult?

Review the physical and psychological preparation of a child for surgery. Review the physical and psychological care of an adult for surgery. Consider that the child generally receives sedation and analgesia before stressful procedures, such as intravenous access. Weigh the developmental needs of a child versus an adult, the child's ability to understand, and so on.

4. How should you prioritize nursing interventions for the client as he wakes from the anesthetic?

Review the immediate postoperative care of a child undergoing surgery. Consider the type of surgery performed, need for positioning, awakening in an unfamiliar environment, and so on. List anticipated problems, such as pain, anxiety, and disorientation. Prioritize your care, considering safety needs first.

5. If you were the client's parent or guardian, what would you need to know before taking the client home?

Think of the questions you might have if the client was your child. Consider information about pain, vomiting, signs of bleeding, signs of infection, food and fluid intake, fever, and so on. Make a list of questions that you feel must be answered prior to taking the client home.

6. How will the client's parent know if he is developing postoperative bleeding?

Research signs and symptoms associated with post-tonsillectomy bleeding. such as frequent clearing of the throat or swallowing, vomiting of bright red blood, restlessness, increased pulse rate, and so on.

7. What attitude or cognitive critical thinking skills did you use to address this case?

Clarification, basic support, reasoning, intellectual empathy, and so on.

Nursing Care of Children

Third-Degree Burns

The client is a 6-year-old girl admitted 4 weeks ago with the diagnosis of third-degree burns covering 90% of her body. She was the victim of a house fire that killed her mother and only sibling. The client was intubated and placed on a ventilator. She now has a temporary tracheostomy, which is suctioned as needed and results in thick yellow-white secretions. She receives around-the-clock rehabilitation protocols. Wound and graft care is extensive for her face, neck, right arm and elbow, right knee, and back. The burns have disfigured her face. In addition, she has undergone partial amputations of both lower extremities. Her nurses apply silver sulfadine lotion to all of her uncovered skin.

She is shy with roommates and tends to be withdrawn. She is aware that her mother and brother died in the fire.

~~~~

1. What are the client's chances for recovery?

   Review the problems associated with extensive third-degree burns, especially for a 6-year-old child. Consider fluid status, electrolyte status, nutrition, activity, the emotional impact of the loss of her mother and brother, and so on. Speculate about factors that may enhance the client's chances for survival and recovery, such as meticulous care of her dressings, management of her wounds, and monitoring of her fluid status.

2. Why is the client at increased risk for developing an infection?

   Explore the risks involved with massive loss of the first line of defense. Consider the presence of invasive central lines, open wounds, her tracheostomy, potential nosocomial infections, and so on. Discuss how trauma of this magnitude impacts the immune response.

3. What is the relationship between the client's fluid and electrolyte status and her burns?

Review the pathophysiological changes that occur from burns, including the seepage of plasma and potential for hypovolemia and hypovolemic shock. Explain how electrolytes are altered when plasma is lost. Identify the electrolytes that are most likely to be affected.

4. What interventions can you implement to help the client deal with the deaths of her mother and brother?

Review interventions for anxiety, stress, and grieving. Reflect on your personal experiences with grief or loss. Identify factors that were helpful and not helpful with the grieving process. Consider whether the client has close relatives or friends that can assist with her care and grief process.

5. How might you feel if you were in the client's situation?

Reflect on your own childhood and the importance you placed on your mother and being like your friends. Discuss with your peers how you might feel about your losses.

6. What attitude and cognitive critical thinking skills did you use when addressing this case?

Divergent thinking, reflection, creativity, intellectual empathy, and so on.

Nursing Care of Children
Traumatic Closed Brain Injury

The client is a 16-year-old male who received a traumatic closed brain injury during an automobile accident a month and a half ago. During his initial hospitalization, the client underwent a splenectomy and tracheostomy, in addition to treatment of his brain injury. Subsequently, the client suffered pleural effusions and infections caused by α-hemolytic Streptococcus and Pseudomonas. The client's mother is his primary caregiver. His father drives a truck for a large company and is away from home at least four nights each week.

Currently, the client is hospitalized in a pediatric subacute-care hospital, undergoing further treatment for his injuries and complications. The client's condition has remained stable. His cardiac status and oxygen saturation levels are being monitored. He is receiving oxygen through a face mask over his tracheostomy. He has required suctioning every 2 to 3 hours but is developing an effective cough on his own as his level of consciousness increases. His health care team is discussing the possibility of removing his tracheostomy tube.

The client's propensity to lose weight resulted in seven diet changes over the past month. He is now receiving 500 mL of extra-strength nutritional supplement over $1^1/2$ hours, five times a day through his gastrostomy tube. His nurses weighed him every Monday and Thursday. A physical therapist performs passive range-of-motion exercises twice daily and assists the client to a chair every day. The client naps frequently, but when awake, he is able to respond to his caregivers' instructions. Over the past several weeks the motion of all his extremities has improved.

On admission, the client scored a 3 out of 14 on the Glasgow Coma Scale with inconsistent responses to "yes" and "no" questions. A radio at his bedside plays music that he likes. Recently the client shed tears when he viewed himself in a mirror. His mother visits every morning and his girlfriend visits whenever possible. He listens to his mother and smiles when she visits. Presently, the health care team is planning a home discharge for the client.

Upon examination, the client is awake and able to respond by shaking his head "yes" and "no" when questioned. His vital signs are within normal limits for his age. He is 5 ft, 10 in tall and weighs 61 kg. He responds to particular stimuli with movements which are not as sporadic or unintentional as they were upon admission. His vital signs are within normal limits for his age, including a regular heart rhythm. His lungs are clear bilaterally, and he has no peripheral edema.

The client's diagnostic findings are within normal limits.

~~~~

1. What does the client's Glasgow Coma Scale mean?

   Review the categories and scoring of the Glasgow Coma Scale. Discuss the meaning of each category. Describe the client on the basis on his last score of 3 out of 14. Consider what can be expected of the client on the basis of his functional ability and level of consciousness.

2. Why was the radio placed at the client's bedside, playing music that he enjoys?

   Discuss the need for and benefits associated with use of voice, music, television, and tape recorders to help overcome sensory deprivation, maintain usual day and night patterns, enrich the environment, and provide familiar input.

3. What preparations will the client's mother have to make in order to take him home?

   Identify and prioritize the client's problems. Speculate about how the client's mother will prepare to address each problem. For example, because the client has difficulty with ambulation and cannot provide his own care, his mother will need to obtain assistive devices to help him move. She may need hospital equipment at home, and he may require daily visits from a home health care aide to assist with the client's hygienic needs, and so on. Consider the client's inability to communicate, decreased mobility, tracheostomy care, tube feedings, and so forth.

4. What risk factors predispose the client to the development of infection?

   Review your list of prioritized problems. Note those factors that predispose the client to infection. Consider his tracheostomy stoma that will not be healed when he arrives home; his gastrostomy tube insertion site; and his splenectomy. Discuss reasons that having a splenectomy alters a person's ability to fight infection.

5. Why is it important to maintaining the client's physical therapy program at home?

   Review the general hazards of immobility. Examine the benefits of passive and active exercises in the maintenance of joint mobility and muscle tone. Discuss the relationship between exercise and muscle strength, pulmonary function, gastrointestinal function, and intestinal mobility. Relate the benefits of exercise to the client's present condition.

6. What concerns may the home health nurse have regarding the client's mother?

   Discuss the burdens and responsibilities of caring for a physically and mentally impaired adolescent at home. Consider her potential for physical and psychological strain and the nursing diagnosis of Caregiver Role Strain. Consider the state of the mother's health, her physical ability to care for her son, and the impact of the father's absence on both the mother and the client.

7. What problems may the client encounter at home as a result of his impaired verbal and nonverbal communication ability?

   Consider how you might feel if you were attempting to communicate your needs and could not be understood. Reflect on your frustration when you cannot understand what a client is trying to communicate. Discuss the emotions that the client and his mother may experience, such as anger, frustration, despair, and so on. Consider the consequences of having an inability to communicate, such as decreased control of the environment or situation and decreased hope of recovery.

8. What community resources might benefit the client and his mother?

   Investigate community service organizations, home health agencies, and health care facilities in your area. Consider referrals to home health nurses, home health aides, physical therapists, occupational therapists, and so on. Describe the benefits of approaching agencies or church members to stay with the client so that the mother can leave the home and spend time alone, do necessary shopping, go to church, and so forth.

9. What critical thinking skills did you use to address the problems presented in this case?

   Divergent thinking, reflection, creativity, intellectual perseverance, and so on.

Mental Health Nursing

The client, a 17-year-old female, has been on the adolescent mental health unit for 2 days. This is her first hospitalization. She has a recent history of truancy, and a history of acting out in school and home. However, she has no substance abuse history. Her parents separated 6 months ago. Since her admission, the client has refused to attend any assigned group activities. She has complained that she has been "incarcerated" against her will. The client's mother admitted her to the hospital after the client hit her and went on a rampage, tearing up things in the house. Her mother called the police for assistance. Since her admission, her father has not visited or called her.

It is the evening shift and you are on the telephone. You hear a scream coming from the lounge and then a crash. You and three other staff members hurry to the lounge and find the client throwing books. Two other clients run out of the room. The nurse-manager decides that the client needs to be physically restrained.

~~~~

1. What is your initial impression of the client's behavior?

   List the thoughts you had about the client's behavior as you read the case. Decide which of your impressions is supported by the data and which are based on first impressions or past experiences. Determine if the data support illness or a difficult adolescent period.

2. What further data are needed to support your impressions?

Review your list of thoughts from question 1. Decide what further data are needed to support your impressions, such as psychological testing; more information from the client about her feelings, especially when she is truant; any drug usage; her relations with her peers; her reaction to her parents' separation, and so on. Consider the need for further discussion with her parents about family events that may be affecting the client.

3. What are the client's priority nursing diagnoses?

Research nursing diagnoses that would be appropriate for the client. Decide if the defining characteristics of the nursing diagnoses you selected fit the client's needs. Focus on nursing diagnoses that address her behavior and safety, as well as the safety of others.

4. How can you best intervene to protect the client and other patients?

Using your textbook or the Nursing Interventions Classification (NIC), research nursing interventions that are most appropriate for the nursing diagnoses you identified. Consider nursing activities, such as separating her from others, use of de-escalation strategies, and so on.

5. On the basis of her behavior, should the client be hospitalized?

Discuss the benefits and disadvantages of hospitalization. Identify behavior manifestations that may warrant hospitalization. Consider the issues surrounding the use of physical restraints on children and adolescents. Discuss inappropriate hospitalization for this age group during the past 5 to 10 years. Research recent court cases and congressional hearings on psychiatric adolescent hospitalization and discuss your findings with your peers.

6. What are the advantages of delaying decisions about the client until all the facts are available?

   Consider the need to refrain from making judgments about children and adolescent psychiatric illness until adequate data are obtained. Discuss the need for adequate information before accurate judgments can be made about any client regardless of the situation.

7. What critical thinking attitudes and skills did you use to address this case?

   Faith in reasoning, reflection, reasoning, basic support, and so on.

Mental Health Nursing
Adolescent Depression

The client is a 17-year-old young woman who is a client in an acute care mental health unit. She was admitted to the hospital 2 days ago for depression and suicidal expressions. She is presently undergoing evaluation. The client vacillates between acknowledging her suicidal feelings and denying them.

A nursing student has been with the client most of the morning. The client approaches the student and asks if the student can keep a secret. The student does not say that she can keep the secret but asks the client to disclose the secret. The client tells the student that she has 20 sleeping pills hidden in her hospital room. She continues to tell the student how important it is for her to be able to trust someone and stresses that the student is helping her by keeping this secret. This is the student's first day on the psychiatric unit. The student believes she has established a successful relationship with the client and is concerned about doing anything to alter the client's feelings of trust.

~~~~

1. If you were this student, what would you do?

   Imagine yourself in this situation and consider your actions. Discuss the advantages of seeking assistance and discuss the consequences of not obtaining help with this problem.

2. What is the most therapeutic way to intervene in this case?

   Review the concept of therapeutic intervention. Identify interventions that would be therapeutic to the client, such as being direct about not being able to keep a secret when safety is concerned and informing the staff without leaving the client alone.

3. Does the client's secret imply that she is planning on taking the pills?

Discuss the need to assume that the client does intend to take the pills and the danger in assuming otherwise. Consider that the client's confidence in you may be a request for help and the client may be hoping that you care enough to intervene. Consider the need to place the client on suicidal precautions.

4. How do you feel about the need to search the client's room?

Identify your feelings about this intrusion of privacy, as well as the possible reaction from the client. Discuss the need for ensuring client safety, even when intrusion of privacy is necessary. Describe the need for conducting a calm, routine search in order to prevent embarrassment for the client. Consider the impact of hospital policies and procedure related to searches.

5. Why does the client vacillate between acknowledging her suicidal feelings and denying them?

Compare the client's behavior with the textbook picture of a person who is depressed and thinking about suicide. Note the characteristic signs that may indicate suicidal thoughts. Discuss the implications of the client making a decision, one way or the other.

6. Do you think that the client's relationship with you will be damaged if you do not keep the secret?

Describe the nurse-client relationship and the need for trust, confidentiality, and so on. Compare the need to protect the client's safety with the need to respect her confidentiality. Consider that you did not promise to keep her secret, as well as your inability to keep a client completely safe.

7. What cognitive and attitude critical thinking skills did you use to address this case?

Intellectual empathy, reflection, basic support, clarification, and so on.

Mental Health Nursing
Anorexia Nervosa

The client, a 15-year-old young woman, was admitted by her pediatrician for evaluation. Her parents, who are divorced, came with her to the hospital. The client lives with her mother and has no siblings. She has no past psychiatric history or other medical problems. Her pediatrician and her parents report that the client has lost 40 lbs in the last year. Despite this weight loss, she has continued to go to school and to excel academically. She also jogs 2 hours every day regardless of the weather conditions. The client has a limited social life.

While the client is an underweight 15-year-old, she appears much younger due to her small body size and development. She is 5 ft, 4 in tall and weighs 90 lb. She carefully removes her shoes, socks, and all outer clothing prior to weighing. She is most concerned about accuracy. The client denies dizziness or seizures. Sometimes she has constipation. She has not had her period in 5 months, but she is not concerned about this change. Upon physical examination, her hands and feet are cold and dry with lanugo on her legs.

The client is defiant during the assessment interview. When she is asked to describe herself, she says that she is overweight. When asked about her typical diet, she responds, "It is normal." She would give no details about her diet. The client wears a large shirt that hangs down to her knees. During the interview, she tells you that she must unpack and will not answer questions unless she can unpack. You notice that she carefully arranges all of her clothing and personal items.

When you interview her mother and father, they say that their daughter will not talk about her weight loss with them. Her mother is well-dressed and thin. She was unaware that her daughter had not had a period for 5 months. The client sees her father once a month. Both parents say that their daughter must have a physical problem that is causing the weight loss. In addition, they think that exercise is important, and they both participate in daily exercise programs.

After the client's first day in the hospital, she has only been out of her room for required activities and has missed some of those. She has not been eating but has been drinking water and orange juice at specific times. You found her exercising in her room, and she refused to stop. The treatment team is meeting to plan further assessments, laboratory testing, and treatments. Her admission diagnosis is anorexia nervosa.

The client's diagnostic findings are as follows:

Vital Signs: Blood pressure 100/70, respirations 20, oral temperature 99.2F, heart rate 82 bpm

Hematology: RBC 3.5, Hgb 10 g/dL, Hct 32%, WBC 4000

Urinalysis: normal

Urine drug screen: negative for illicit drugs

~~~~

1. What further data do you need regarding the client's physical status?

   Review the need for a thorough physical assessment of a client suspected of having anorexia nervosa. Discuss the need to assess this person's weight; menstrual cycle; cardiac, gastrointestinal, dental, renal, and endocrine status; eating habits, body image, self-esteem, mental status, and so on. Explain the relationship between symptoms such as seizures, peripheral edema, heart palpitations, sore throat, loss of teeth, and the presence of anorexia.

2. What data support the inference that the client is suffering from an eating disorder?

   Separate the data into relevant subjective and objective categories. Review the common clinical manifestations of anorexia nervosa. Compare the client's subjective and objective data with the clinical manifestations of anorexia described in your textbook. Consider the client's weight loss, physical appearance, clothing, few friends, academic achievement, obsession with exercise, need for order, and so on.

3. How are anorexia nervosa and bulimia different?

Research the conditions of anorexia nervosa and bulimia. Compare and contrast the two conditions on the basis of their etiologies or precipitating factors, environmental and sociocultural factors, and clinical manifestations and their consequences. Discuss these disorders from the perspective of neurobiological theory.

4. What are the relationships between body image, need for control, and eating disorders?

Discuss the possible impact of altered body image on food intake. Explain how the need for control can alter a person's food intake.

5. What do you think is the most likely communication style of this family on the basis of the data provided?

Discuss the importance of family dynamics in the client's recovery. Consider the parents' divorce, mutual concern about body image, their lack of awareness about the client's menstrual cycle, and so on. Describe the family's communication style on the basis of your assessment of the family dynamics.

6. What are the priority nursing diagnoses for the client?

On the basis of your understanding of anorexia, identify nursing diagnoses that address actual and potential physiologic and psychologic problems. Describe the client's possible adaptive and maladaptive responses to her eating disorder. Consider nursing diagnoses that address altered body image, disturbed self-esteem, physiologic complications related to altered intake, malnutrition or starvation, excessive exercise, and so on.

7. How can you best address the nursing diagnoses you identified?

   Identify nursing interventions that address each of your nursing diagnoses. Consider interventions that address nutritional stabilization, body image, control issues, consistent procedures for daily weights, group activities, education about anxiety and depression, family therapy, goal setting for specific weight outcomes, and so on. Discuss the critical need for consistency and limit setting related to excessive exercise and inadequate food intake.

8. What are your biases about adolescents such as the client?

   Identify the feelings that you experienced when you read this case. Decide if you have positive or negative biases about eating disorders. Identify overt and subtle pressures that you have experienced related to body image. Reflect on your personal experiences with dieting and explain how your past experiences with dieting or body image impact your present feelings.

9. What should you include during discharge planning for the client?

   Discuss the client's home environment where she will return. Consider follow-up therapy, diet and exercise control, social activities, her return to school, signs indicating a relapse to former behaviors, and so forth.

10. What attitude and cognitive critical thinking skills did you use when answering the questions regarding the client?

   Clarification, reasoning, reflection, intellectual empathy, and so on.

Mental Health Nursing
Antisocial Personality Disorder

The client is a 17-year-old young man who has been described as a troubled child since the age of 7 or 8. He has a long history of fighting with other students; biting his classmates; stealing from his peers, parents, or siblings; and repeated shoplifting and stealing in his community. He has been caught and prosecuted on two occasions, one of which resulted in his father paying a large fine and the other resulted in 6 months of probation.

The client has held a couple of low-paying jobs, but he was terminated for aggressive behavior or suspicion of stealing. He consistently denies any wrong-doing, makes excuses for his behavior, or blames someone else for his failure. When confronted about his behavior, the client fails to show remorse for having broken the law or for physically or emotionally hurting others.

Most recently, the client was caught breaking and entering into an apartment building. His parents have admitted the client to the hospital because they realize they can no longer control his behavior and fear that his recent crime will result in a prison sentence.

~~~~~

1. What conclusions can you draw about the client on the basis of his present situation and past behavior?

   Cluster the data into related categories. Identify patterns within and between the data clusters. Consider the possibility that the client has borderline personality disorder or antisocial personality disorder. Discuss the need for further information before you can draw accurate conclusions.

2. What further data are needed to support your conclusions?

Review the data that support your conclusions about the client's diagnosis, including characteristics that appeared before age 15, such as his lying, stealing, fighting, and aggression; his inability to sustain employment or relationships; his lack of guilt or concern for others, and so on. Research antisocial personality disorder and decide what further data are needed to diagnose the client with this condition, such as results of psychological testing, more information about his home life, behavior patterns of his siblings, the type of parenting he experienced, the relationship between his parents, and so on.

3. How can you explain the client's behavior from the context of social causative theory?

Research social causative theory. Compare the client's clinical manifestations with those presented in the textbook. Consider the client's personality trait that places himself and his needs before those of others or society, his need for immediate gratification, and so on. Discuss how you can explain his behavior using this theory.

4. How can caring for this client help you care for clients experiencing borderline personality disorder?

Discuss the similarities in the two disorders, for example, clients may exhibit similar characteristics, such as aggression, manipulation, inability to accept responsibility, inability to care for or love others, and so on. Decide if interventions for the client would help clients with borderline personality disorder, such as using a consistent, straightforward, and businesslike approach; providing group therapy; planning small steps together toward achieving therapeutic goals; and setting limits on destructive behaviors.

5. What are your personal biases about this case?

   Identify your feelings as you read about the client. Consider whether your feelings reflect a positive or negative bias about clients with personality disorders. Reflect on your experiences that helped shape your feelings or biases. Explain why it is important to identify your own biases when planning care for clients such as this young man.

6. What attitude and cognitive critical thinking skills did you use to address this case?

   Intellectual humility, reflection, reasoning, divergent thinking, and so on.

Mental Health Nursing
Anxiety and Panic Attacks

The client was admitted to the mental health unit with a diagnosis of anxiety with panic attacks. For the last 6 months, she has been experiencing panic attacks and severe anxiety for which she has not sought treatment. The client would not leave her home and was unable to work for the last month. She has no past psychiatric history or other medical problems.

Her partner convinced her to go to the emergency department when he returned from work and found her sitting on the floor in the corner of their bedroom covered in urine. She had been too frightened to leave the corner all day. He told the emergency department nurse that they have been happily married for the past 3 years. His wife is a successful interior decorator. She had been under considerable stress when her major client decided to discontinue his contract. The only medication she had taken was oral contraceptives, and he could not remember the name of the medication. After further consultation with her partner, the health care team decided to hospitalize the client.

The client, a 35-year-old woman, was admitted in soiled clothes. She appeared frightened. Her hands moved constantly, and she paced in one area. Directions had to be repeated several times for her to comprehend. She cooperated with the admission process as long as she could pace. To alleviate her anxiety, the nurse administered 3 mg of lorazepam intramuscularly. Her heart rate was 92 beats per minute (bpm), her blood pressure was 140/90, her respirations were 30, and her oral temperature was 98.6F.

The client's diagnostic findings are as follows:

Urine Drug Screen: negative for illicit drugs

Hematology: RBC 4.2, Hgb 12 g/dL, Hct 38%, WBC 5000

Following 3 days of hospitalization and medication with a 2-mg tablet of lorazepam twice a day, the client became more cooperative with treatment, attended group therapy, and socialized with other clients. The nurse assigned to the client wants to help her learn more about anxiety and stress reduction. She sets up a time to talk with the client about these topics, as well as her discharge. The client will be discharged in 2 days. She is, however, becoming anxious about the discharge and is demanding to know why she cannot stay longer. The nurse explains that her insurance will only cover a 5-day hospitalization.

~~~~

1. What data support the nursing and medical diagnosis of anxiety?

   Review the clinical manifestations of anxiety. Compare such manifestations with data regarding the client. Identify assessments and related parameters to monitor the degree of the client's anxiety.

2. What is the relationship between the client's anxiety and panic attacks and the stress of her job?

   Review the concept of pathologic anxiety and factors that cause or accelerate anxiety, such as high stress, little or no time for relaxation, anxiety related to failure, and low self-esteem.

3. How can the nurse help the client reduce her stress and, thus, reduce her anxiety?

   Review methods for stress and anxiety reduction. Decide which method would benefit the client, such as problem-solving with her to find a way to decrease her workload, suggesting stress-reduction techniques, and so on.

4. Formulate an education plan for the client regarding anxiety.

   Review pertinent elements of a client education plan for anxiety. Decide which elements are most appropriate for the client on the basis of the information you have. Consider issues such as symptom monitoring, relaxation and stress management, social activities, follow-up psychotherapy, problem solving, supportive strategies for the client's partner, and so on.

5. Why is the client concerned about her discharge?

   Consider whether all clients are pleased to be discharged from the hospital. Discuss client needs that hospitalization may address. Identify possible concerns and fears that the client may have about loss of security and support that hospitalization offered. Consider her possible fear of relapse, the stigma of hospitalization that she may face from friends or acquaintances, her ability to handle the stress of personal life and work, and so on.

6. What nursing interventions should be considered to assist the client with discharge?

   Identify interventions designed to reduce stress and lower anxiety, such as using relaxation techniques, providing clear discharge plans that include both the client and her partner, scheduling a follow-up appointment, providing phone numbers to call for help, and so on. Discuss the need for the client to verbalize her fears and to discuss what she thinks will happen when she goes home.

7. What impact may the client's short hospitalization have on her progress?

   Weigh the advantages and disadvantages of shorter hospitalization on clients with mental health problems. Discuss the need for avoiding overt criticism of the client's insurance company which could increase her anxiety.

8. How are you affected by your own anxieties?

   Reflect on your past experiences and identify anxiety-producing conditions. Discuss anxiety as a normal reaction that everyone experiences. Identify the degree of anxiety that produces an abnormal reaction, such as mild, moderate, severe, and panic levels of anxiety. Consider the consequences of prolonged anxiety, such as increased likelihood of developing problems that will require interventions. Explain the importance of assessing your own anxiety and knowing when to seek assistance.

9. What attitude and cognitive critical thinking skills did you use to address this case?

Clarification, reasoning, reflection, intellectual empathy, and so on.

Mental Health Nursing
Delusional Behavior

The client is a 45-year-old man who is single and lives alone. He has a close relationship with his parents, ages 70 and 75, and his younger sister, age 40. All of his family live in the same city. The client is employed as a teller at a local bank. While at work, he became disruptive, unable to work, and unable to control his angry outbursts. Bank officials summoned the police who took him to the emergency department. The health care workers notified his sister.

The client was incoherent upon arrival at the hospital. His sister provided his medical history, which included diabetes mellitus controlled by daily insulin, no known allergies, and weight loss within the last few weeks. The sister described her brother as social, except for occasional periods during which he appeared to be "high" and "on the move," rambling and unable to concentrate. She described times when he was "down," lost weight, and had problems with his diabetes. He shocked the family last week when he purchased a new car that he did not need. Two days ago, he announced that he was quitting his job for a better one. The client has never been treated for a mental illness, and his family is concerned about his recent behavior. Because the client is not cooperative and repeatedly attempts to run out of the examining room screaming, the nurses have employed physical restraints.

The client is uncooperative with the physical examination, but he is able to answer some questions coherently. His speech is rapid, rambling, and anxious. He frequently states that he needs to go home and sleep. He appears tired, with circles under his eyes, and he is sweating. His clothing fits loosely, but he is clean and dressed appropriately. He is unable to maintain eye contact for more than 3 seconds and alternates between yelling and speaking in a normal tone of voice, laughing inappropriately and being belligerent. At times, his responses are incongruent with his speech. He denies that he is having problems, stating that his diabetes has been cured and his life is perfect. He also denies hallucinations but believes that he needed to quit his job because he had become president of the bank.

He is oriented to person, place, and time but demonstrates flight of ideas and is, at times, unable to answer questions. His remote, recent, and immediate memory are intact. He is unable to concentrate or calculate. He verbalizes no insight into his illness, repeating that he focuses on his perfect health, life, and new position.

He is 5 ft, 9 in tall and weighs 145 lbs. His usual weight, according to his sister, is 160 lbs. His blood pressure is 140/90, his heart rate is 95 beats per minute (bpm), his respirations are 25 breaths per minute, and his oral temperature is 98.7F.

The client's diagnostic findings are as follows:

Blood glucose: 25 mg/dL

Urinalysis: positive for glucose and ketones

Urine drug screen: negative for illicit drugs

~~~~

1. What can you infer from the data regarding the client?

   Group the data into subjective and objective categories. Identify patterns within and between the categories of data. Identify problems or nursing diagnoses that are appropriate for data clusters. Speculate about the possible causes of the client's current behavior on the basis of his medical history and present blood glucose levels. Consider whether the client is exhibiting symptoms of bipolar disorder and is manic at this time.

2. What are the possible consequences of placing someone such as the client in physical restraints?

   Compare the advantages and disadvantages of using physical restraints. Identify behavior patterns that may be aggravated by the use of restraints. Consider the physical risks imposed by restraints, especially with a diabetic client, for example, nutritional and fluid needs, loss of fluids through perspiration, toileting, injuries to skin, and so on. Identify important monitoring and assessment parameters for the client in restraints, including frequency of assessments and factors to assess when restraints are removed.

3. How does the use of physical restraints impact a client's rights?

Discuss client's rights and how the use of physical restraints may infringe on those rights. Discuss alternatives to using physical restraints. Present instances in which use of physical restraint is essential. Identify data that suggest that physical restraints may be necessary in this case.

4. What outcomes would you want for the person who must be treated with restraints?

Discuss the importance of formulating desired outcomes as early in the care process as possible. Research documentation requirements when restraints are used. Explain why hospitals have policies regarding use of and documentation about use of restraints. Discuss the need for carefully following physician orders and institutional policies. Use the Nursing Outcomes Classification (NOC) to identify appropriate outcomes for the client.

5. How do you feel about the use of physical restraints?

Image how you would feel if someone physically restrained you. Examine your feelings and discuss those feelings with a peer. Identify any conditions under which you believe restraints would be appropriate, such as an unsafe situation for the health care worker. Discuss whether you believe restraints are used indiscriminately or too often. As a nurse, think about what you can do to ensure appropriate use of physical restraints.

6. How are the client's blood glucose level and his current behavior related?

Review the pathophysiology of hyperglycemia and ketoacidosis. Discuss clinical manifestations that occur with uncontrolled hyperglycemia. Compare those signs and symptoms with the client's clinical presentation. Discuss the impact of the client's bipolar disorder, especially this period of mania, on his ability to appropriately follow dietary guidelines, which is critical for the diabetic client. Explain how altered blood glucose levels can affect behavior in any person, not just those with mental disorders.

7. Why does the client have little or no insight into his current situation?

Explore the impact of physical and mental illness on the ability to view yourself insightfully. Discuss the degree of physical or mental health that is necessary for a person to have insight.

8. How are hallucinations similar to and different from delusions and which is the client experiencing?

Review the clinical manifestations of hallucinations and delusions. Identify data that suggest that the client is hallucinating or having delusions. Assess factors in the client's present situation that may be contributing to his delusions.

9. What nursing interventions should take priority in this case?

Discuss the use of the Nursing Interventions Classification (NIC) to assist you in planning care for the client. Review data obtained in question 1 and select interventions most appropriate for the priority problems you identified. Consider interventions that address hyperglycemia, delusions, and so on.

10. What critical thinking skills did you use to answer the questions pertaining to this case?

Reflection, intellectual perseverance, basic support, clarification, and so on.

Mental Health Nursing
Depression

The client, a 67-year-old man, was admitted to the mental health unit 2 days ago for a short evaluation of his depression. His wife, who initiated the admission, states that the client has never been diagnosed with or treated for depression. He has, however, exhibited symptoms of depression over the past year. She decided to admit the client to the hospital because he stated on several occasions that he was going to kill himself. The claims adjuster from the client's insurer has informed the hospital that the client cannot remain hospitalized longer than 5 days.

After performing a diagnostic evaluation, the client's physician determined that he has major depression. The client is placed on 15 mg of the medication phenelzine sulfate twice a day. The hospital staff expects him to attend the Medication Education Group. Attempting to avoid the meeting, the client stays in his room, and a staff member has to find him and escort him to the meeting. The client thinks that he needs to just take the medication and his depression will quickly subside. With prompting, he introduces himself to the group, stating, "These pills are like any other pills."

~~~~

1. What data, other than the client's threats of suicide, indicate depression?

   Review the pathology of depression. Describe clinical manifestations that are common to various degrees of depression. Identify the stage of depression when suicidal ideation is most likely to occur.

2. Do you think the client's wife made the right decision about admitting him to the psychiatric unit?

Discuss the degree of depression that must be present before a person talks about suicide. Explain the purpose behind threatening suicide. Reflect on past experiences with other depressed or suicidal clients. Make a judgment about the client's wife's decision on the basis of the limited amount of information provided.

3. How will you know if the medication phenelzine sulfate is effective?

Investigate the medication phenelzine sulfate, noting its intended actions and its side effects. Discuss the length of time it takes to achieve therapeutic levels so that its actions can be evaluated. Identify changes that will occur in the client's demeanor if the medication is effective.

4. What is the relationship between the client's reluctance to participate with the group and his state of depression?

Discuss how depression affects behavior, communication, social interactions, and the ability to cope with others. Consider the need for more information, for example, did the client enjoy group activities prior to his illness? Describe how depression can change a person's personality.

5. What are the client's priority nursing diagnoses?

Review nursing diagnoses that apply to the depressed client. After reviewing the defining characteristics of the diagnosis, decide if they appropriate for the client's circumstances. Address his mental needs, physical needs, and care giver's needs.

6. What interventions are most appropriate for the client at this time?

   Research interventions that address the nursing diagnoses you identified. Consider the need for client education about depression and about prescribed medications; the need for one-to-one discussion about his concerns and fears, such as the fear that he might harm himself so he needs treatments that work quickly or his fear that the depression will not subside; and discussion about this reaction to his diagnosis and treatment. Consider the need to discuss his insurance benefits and the possible treatment constraints that his insurance or financial status may impose.

7. What are the possible consequences or advantages of the client's brief hospitalization?

   Discuss the current trend toward short hospitalizations. Consider the advantages of quickly returning to a familiar environment. Identify the possible consequences of discharging the client before his medications are fully effective, especially when suicidal ideation is present.

8. What assessments should you make prior to discharging the client to go home?

   Discuss the need for a complete assessment to determine nursing diagnoses and accurate etiologies. Consider the client's present physical and mental status, including his suicidal ideation, safety needs, and so on. Assess the appropriateness of his treatment plan. Determine his ability to comply with treatment recommendations, including medications and follow-up care. Consider assessing his family's reaction to this illness and discharge to home.

9. What critical thinking skills or attitudes did you use to address this case?

   Intellectual courage, basic support, clarification, creativity, and so on.

Mental Health Nursing
Depression and Suicidal Ideation

The client is a 60-year-old woman whose physician ordered home health nursing for her following a 5-day admission to the acute care hospital with a medical diagnosis of major depression and suicidal ideation. She lives with her 75-year-old partner. They have no children. This was her first admission for depression and her first referral for home care. The physician orders include 35 mg of fluoxetine hydrochloride per day and assessment of the client's adjustment to home. She has no other medical problems but has lost 35 lbs in the last 6 months.

The client does not greet the nurse when she arrives. When introduced by her partner, the client tells the nurse, "I don't need any help; I know what to do." The client's partner adds that his wife has taken the medication as the physician prescribed. The client appears to be older than her age of 60. She is neatly dressed but appears tired and eager to have the nurse leave. She answers some of the questions but supplies only short answers. She refuses to discuss suicidal thoughts, informing the nurse that it is none of her business. Her only complaints are of dry mouth and occasional dizziness. Her partner seems concerned. He tells the nurse at the door that his wife just does not seem right, but he is pleased that she dressed herself. She seems to have more energy even though she looks tired.

The client is 5 ft, 6 in and weighs 107 lbs, which was her weight at the time of discharge from the hospital. Her blood pressure is 110/70, her heart rate is 88 beats per minute (bpm), her respirations are 20 breaths per minute, and her oral temperature is 98.7F.

Laboratory test results from hospitalization are within normal ranges. Her physician has not ordered any further tests.

~~~~

1. What further assessment data are needed to determine the seriousness of the client's suicidal intentions?

   Consider the data related to changes in her behavior, her partner's observations, your observations, feelings she has shared with her partner, and so on. Decide if you have data to indicate she has a plan to commit suicide. Consider whether she has a means to harm herself.

2. Does the data support a high or low risk of suicide?

   Cluster the data into categories that support high risk versus low risk of suicide. Consider the client's increased energy, ability to dress herself, compliance with her medication regimen, tired appearance, refusal to discuss suicidal feelings, and so on.

3. What is the relationship between increased energy in a depressed patient and the risk of suicide?

   Review the clinical manifestations that forewarn of suicide. Discuss the need for energy in order to plan or attempt suicide. Research the incidence of suicide among individuals who were thought to be improving.

4. Which nursing diagnoses take precedence in this case?

   Review diagnoses by the North American Nursing Diagnosis Association (NANDA) related to depression and suicide. Decide if the defining characteristics fit the data given for the client. Prioritize the diagnoses you selected according to the life-preservation framework or another prioritizing framework provided by your school. On the basis of your prioritizations, determine the most important nursing diagnosis.

5. What nursing activities can you implement to address the client's intentions?

Describe the advantages of using a treatment or "no harm" contract, written with the client and her partner. Discuss the need to explain the treatment contract, including its purpose and development. Explain the role of the client's partner and the concept of partnership concerning the treatment contract. Clarify the client's and her partner's role in the home with concrete examples, such as teaching, providing proper nutrition, practicing stress management, and so on. Discuss the importance of goal setting as a nursing-initiated activity. Consider the possibility that the client may view you as a "watchdog."

6. What further data are needed to determine the source of the client's partner's concerns?

Identify behaviors that another person may interpret as suicidal. Consider other factors that may influence the client's partner, such as changes in the client's behavior, certain expressions of thoughts or feelings, side effects of medications, the caregiver's own health, the impact of the spouse's illness, and so on.

7. What can you do to ensure that the client and her partner receive appropriate education if they did not receive such information during the client's hospitalization?

Discuss the impact of shorter hospitalizations on client education. Describe the need to assess the couple's knowledge of medications, beginning with side effects because the client is experiencing dry mouth and dizziness. Explain how you could assess the need for further education, the client's tolerance for learning, and the impact of her illness on her learning.

8. How are aging and depression related?

Examine issues of aging, such as financial losses, friends' illnesses or deaths, fears of a spouse's health, reduced activity and social life, absence of children to offer emotional or physical support, and so on. Consider Erikson's last stage of development and its relationship to depression and suicide in the elderly.

9. Can you prevent someone from committing suicide?

Review the pathophysiology of depression and suicidal ideation. Consider whether all suicides can be prevented, even when warning signs and help are available. Discuss the issues of staff guilt and feelings of failure when someone does commit suicide. Consider the idea that no one can be totally protected.

10. What attitude and cognitive critical thinking skills did you use to address the issues in this case?

Divergent thinking, clarification, reflection, intellectual perseverance, and so on.

Mental Health Nursing

Involuntary Hospital Admission for Schizophrenia

The client, a 57-year-old man, voluntarily admitted himself to the hospital. He has a medical diagnosis of schizophrenia. The client has a history of multiple admissions over the past 10 years, often caused by violent behavior toward others. After 2 days in the hospital, the client decides that he wants to leave. He is, however, delusional and threatening to kill his boss at the printing company where he is employed. The client's physician decides that if he continues to insist on leaving, he will have to commit him involuntarily.

The client's wife and daughter are concerned and do not understand what involuntary commitment means. They are extremely upset. The client's wife is crying, and his 25-year-old daughter is demanding an explanation. Responding to his family's emotional state, the client becomes angry, and the three of them demand his immediate release. Other clients on the unit are standing around the nurses' station observing the turmoil.

~~~~

1. What does "involuntary" admission or commitment mean?

    Define the term "involuntary." Investigate the meaning of involuntary admission in your state. Identify the criteria for involuntary admission to a psychiatric facility.

2. Who makes the final decision to involuntarily commit someone to a psychiatric facility?

   Investigate the policies and procedures regarding involuntary commitment of an individual to a psychiatric facility in your area. Investigate state laws regarding such admissions. Identify documentation requirements, time limits, required assessments, and client and family rights, concerning involuntary commitment to a psychiatric facility. Consider the family's need to understand what is happening and what will happen once a person is involuntarily admitted. Discuss both the client's and family's loss of control in such instances.

3. In your opinion, does the client's behavior warrant involuntary admission to the hospital?

   Determine whether the client should be involuntarily admitted. Identify criteria or data that you used to support your opinion, such as client safety, safety of others, the client's ability to recognize his need for help, and so on.

4. How will the client's care differ if he voluntarily agreed to stay in the hospital or if he was admitted involuntarily?

   Review the policies and procedures for hospital admission that require him to remain in a locked area. Explain the treatments for clients who are involuntarily admitted to a psychiatric facility, stressing that care should be no different from that of clients admitted voluntarily.

5. If you were the nurse, how might you react to the family's demands?

   Identify possible reactions that you might have. Reflect on instances in which you have seen clients or families lose control and the effect such instances had on nearby staff and other clients. Discuss other clients' probable fears that the same thing could happen to them.

6. If you support involuntary commitment, how could you argue effectively for the opposite point of view? If you do not support involuntary commitment, how could you argue in favor of committing a client against his will?

   Identify your feelings on this issue. After reaching a conclusion about involuntary commitment, argue for the opposite choice. Consider the criteria that you used to develop your argument. Discuss whether your criteria were based on fact or on emotions. Compare your feelings with those of your classmates.

7. What critical thinking attitudes and skills did you use to address this case?

   Basic support, clarification, reflection, reasoning, intellectual courage, and so on.

Mental Health Nursing
Long-Term Care

The client is a 75-year-old widow who has recently been admitted to a long-term care facility. On admission, the client stated that she did not want to be there and wanted to go back to her own home. Accustomed to hearing such comments from newly admitted residents, the staff members generally ignored the comment and tried to console her. The client refused to eat anything on her first day in the facility. She did not converse with other residents and spent her time alone in her room.

Two weeks later, the client still has not spoken to other residents and continues to stay in her room. She follows directions from staff members but makes no effort to communicate with them otherwise. She picks at her food and eats little. The client appears tired. During a staff team meeting with the psychiatric nurse consultant, staff members complain that they have tried to help the client but are growing tired of her behavior. They express their feelings about being overworked and having better things to do than sit around discussing the client's behavior.

~~~~

1. What can you infer about this situation?

   Identify data that are most relevant to the client's present situation. Cluster the data into categories containing similar information. Identify problems and appropriate nursing diagnoses, considering the client's degree of independence, support systems, and so on. Decide if you can make any inferences on the basis of the data provided.

2. What data would further support your inferences?

Review your inferences regarding the client's condition. Identify missing information that would clarify her current problem, including the client's physical state of health, history or clinical manifestations of depression, and so on.

3. How might you feel if you were in the client's situation?

Reflect on past experiences in which you were required to do something that you did not want to do. Consider conditions that made you feel better or worse. Think about the implications of giving up your independence and having to adjust to a new environment. Speculate about your feelings.

4. What are the client's priority nursing diagnoses from a mental health perspective?

Consider whether the client's reaction is related to her admission to the long-term care facility, depression, or a combination of the two. Identify the client's problems and the most appropriate nursing diagnoses to address them. After selecting the most appropriate nursing diagnoses, prioritize them on the basis of the life-preservation framework or another prioritizing framework provided by your school.

5. What nursing interventions should take priority?

Discuss the impact of mental status changes on physical status. Assess the client's nutritional status and her need for a sleep assessment. Consider gradually increasing her activities on the basis of her interests, allowing her some sense of control over small decisions, conducting an open discussion about her responses, and including her family members in planning sessions.

6. If you were the nurse consultant, how might you respond to the staff members?

Identify several methods for dealing with staff reactions and concerns. Consider that staff members may need education about depression, losses experienced by the elderly, and so on. Assess the staff members' feelings. Consider whether they feel that they have failed, whether they have cared for similar residents in the past, and what interventions were successful. Assess the staff members' reactions and whether they reflect another problem, such as inadequate time with new residents or fatigue and stress from heavy workloads.

7. What critical thinking attitudes and skills did you use to address this case?

Divergent thinking, reasoning, basic support, intellectual empathy, and so on.

Mental Health Nursing
Paranoid Schizophrenia

The client is 35 years old and lives with her parents. From reading the referral information and speaking with her physician, you learn that the client's diagnosis is paranoid schizophrenia. She is unable to work and fears leaving her home. The client was discharged from the local hospital yesterday after a 3-day admission for acute psychosis. She has a long history of noncompliance with medication and multiple hospitalizations since age 22. As a result, she has never been able to hold a full-time job and has worked sporadically in sheltered work-shop settings.

Two months ago, she was discharged from a partial hospitalization program. She had attended this program for 4 months and was attached to the staff. Her discharge occurred because she had met the outcomes identified for her at the time of admission to the partial hospitalization program: ability to relate to others appropriately, compliance with medication and treatment, and ability to communicate appropriately with her parents.

The physician orders for home care include 300 mg of clozapine twice a day. This is your first visit to see the client.

~~~~

1. What assessments are most essential on this first visit with the client?

   Prioritize your assessments for a client with paranoid schizophrenia. Consider assessing her for delusions, hallucinations, medication compliance, possible side effects of medications, ability to problem solve and communicate, and so on.

2. What is your most appropriate reaction if the client is suspicious of your presence?

Discuss language and behaviors that may increase the client's paranoia and the need to avoid those reactions. Consider the benefit derived from avoiding physical touch, maintaining physical distance from the client, using clear communication and avoiding the use of pronouns, avoiding secrets with the family, and allowing the client to set some limits, and so on.

3. What are the advantages of partial hospitalization programs compared to full hospitalization?

Compare the benefits of partial hospitalization with those of full hospitalization. Consider potential advantages to partial hospitalization, such as increased client flexibility and freedom, ability to live with her family while receiving treatment, ability to continue with school or work activities (some programs support gradual transition back to school or work), client support as she reintegrates with the community and her personal life, decreased cost, increased time for client education, and skill development opportunities.

4. How can you support the client's parents?

Research nursing activities that may support family members in this situation, such as providing information and education about schizophrenia; providing uninterrupted time for them to verbalize their concerns despite the paranoid feelings from their daughter, and suggesting support groups that might benefit them. Research community support agencies that are available in your community. Select the most appropriate agencies to assist the client's parents.

5. What teaching do you think you would need if you were one of the client's parents?

   Think about your own knowledge base regarding schizophrenia. Decide what information would be most helpful to you. Consider the need for information about biological aspects of schizophrenia; symptoms that indicate problems and the best methods of monitoring for those symptoms; medication schedules, actions, and side effects; problem-solving strategies; coping strategies for living with the client while allowing time for themselves; strategies for setting limits; and planning for the future, including plans for the client after her parents died, and so on. Discuss how a caregiver's death presents a major problem when the caregiver is a parent and the patient is an adult child.

6. How might you feel if you could not make your needs understood?

   Consider how you might feel if you thought your communications were clear and yet no one could understand you. Discuss the aspects of paranoid schizophrenia that make the client believe that she is not being understood.

7. What attitude and cognitive critical thinking skills did you use to address this case?

   Intellectual empathy, clarification, basic support, reasoning, reflection, and so on.

Mental Health Nursing
Patient-Caregiver Conflict

The client is an 89-year-old woman who recently moved in with her daughter and son-in-law. She was unable to continue living alone due to increasing weakness and forgetfulness. Seven weeks ago, she fell in her bathtub and fractured her left hip. After surgical repair of the hip, she recovered slowly and spent several weeks in a rehabilitation facility. A home health visit was scheduled to assist with the client's adjustment and assess her needs for home health care. The client is alone during the day while her daughter and son-in-law work.

Upon the initial visit, the daughter met you outside and told you, "My mother won't do anything she's supposed to. If the doctor tells her one thing, she does exactly the opposite. She won't eat right, take her medication, or do her exercises. I'm at my wit's end." While you were talking to the client, her daughter interrupted frequently and answered for her mother. She fussed over the client and made her change positions several times. The client became irritated and snapped at her daughter, who then left the room. The client admitted that she didn't always take her medications but responded positively when you explained the actions of the drugs and helped her fill out a medication planner so she could take her medications without help. You also learned that the client believed her daughter was not supporting her rights or her need for independence.

~~~~

1. What are the primary issues in this situation?

   Review the objective and subjective data presented in this case. Identify the priority needs of both the daughter and mother. Determine how those needs may conflict. Consider the daughter's need to protect her mother's welfare, as well as the mother's need to take care of herself as long as possible. Discuss the issue of role reversal when parents become dependent on their children.

2. What inferences about the client's relationship with her daughter can be justified by the data?

   * Discuss your first impressions, such as the client and her daughter are not getting along, the daughter is trying to control her mother, and so on. Consider the impact of a stressful event or illness on the lives of family members and the client's fear regarding loss of independence.

   * Cluster the data into related categories. Decide what inferences you can accurately make on the basis of the data presented. Discuss the need for further information in order to confirm your inferences.

3. How can you best intervene to assist both the client and her daughter?

   Discuss your role as a home health nurse to be a client advocate, care provider, and counselor. Suggest ways for the mother and daughter to resolve their conflict, such as jointly identifying activities for which the client needs assistance and those she can and prefers to do independently.

4. What characteristics does the client display that a younger adult may or may not exhibit?

   Review the case and note factors that may have contributed to the client's reaction, such as feelings of anger, humiliation, or desire for revenge from her daughter. Explore how feelings may be similar regardless of age. Consider that older people may value their independence more than younger people because they know they will soon have to relinquish some, if not all, of that independence.

5. What are the possible consequences to the client or her daughter if you draw conclusions about their relationship before obtaining more data?

Discuss the problems associated with drawing premature conclusions about any issue. Consider the possible consequences of formulating inaccurate conclusions about either the client's or her daughter's motives. Reflect on your past experiences in which someone drew inaccurate, premature conclusions about you. Discuss your feelings at the time and the outcome of that experience.

6. What attitude and cognitive critical thinking skills did you use to answer the questions pertaining to this case?

Divergent thinking, reflection, intellectual humility, faith in reason, and so on.

Potentially Dangerous Home Health Visit

You are working for a home health agency. You have been assigned to a new client, a 50-year-old man who is recovering from surgery and adjusting to a permanent colostomy. You note that the client also has a diagnosis of paranoid schizophrenia but has no history of violent behavior. He is compliant with is medication, 1 mg of haloperidol twice a day. He schedules and keeps regular follow-up appointments at a community mental health clinic, where he receives medication assessments and crisis intervention as needed. The client works part-time for a local landscaping business and lives alone. He has been in stable mental and physical health for the past year. You expect, therefore, that this will be a typical colostomy follow-up visit.

Upon arriving at the client's home, you realize that he will need to have a home health aide for a period of time. While conversing with the client, you see that there is a gun lying on the table next to his chair.

~~~~

1. How should you respond when you note the presence of the gun?

   Discuss the need to remove the gun from the room and possibly the home. Consider whether you should leave immediately if the gun is not removed. Identify the most important consideration in this situation, focusing on safety, and explain your rationale. Reflect on how you might feel if this actually happened to you.

2. Should you consider the client dangerous?

   Discuss the need to consider any client dangerous when a gun is present, emphasizing the need for safety.

3. What further information do you need?

Discuss the need for further information explaining why the gun is present. Assess the client's fears, such as fear for his own safety, and whether his concerns may be justified (living in a high-crime area). Consider the client's potential for suicide, possible paranoid ideation, and so on. Discuss the possible psychological impact of an altered body image related to the colostomy.

4. What are the advantages of delaying any actions or decisions until all the facts are available?

Discuss the possible consequences of drawing incorrect conclusions and acting on incomplete information. Consider how each possible explanation for the gun, including fear for the client's safety and suicidal tendencies may affect his treatment and how premature conclusions may not provide the client with the help he needs.

5. What conditions support the need for a home health aide?

Review the client's data, noting those conditions that support the need for a home health aide, such as the client living alone and needing continued post-operative care, assistance during his adjustment to his new colostomy and change in lifestyle, and further assessment of his mental status.

6. What attitude and cognitive critical thinking skills did you use to address this case?

Divergent thinking, basic support, intellectual humility, faith in reason, and so on.

Mental Health Nursing
Restrained Client

You have just begun to work on an acute care psychiatric unit in a community hospital. During your orientation, you observe that three clients are in four-point restraints in their rooms. You review one of their medical records and find that the client has been in restraints for 30 hours. There is only one order, a verbal one, from the physician, and it was obtained at the time of initial restraint. The documented reason for use of restraints was that the client hit another client while arguing over the television. No staff member observed the interaction. The record further indicates that the client has been in continuous restraints since then.

The notes are sparse about his communication or behavior during the 30 hours he has been restrained. Examples of such documentation include the following:

2200: Client asleep

0900: Client staring into space

You cannot find any comments indicating that a staff member communicated with the client or addressed his physical needs.

~~~~

1. What can you conclude about the restraint of this particular client?

   Discuss the need for further documentation in order to draw accurate conclusions about this client. Using your textbook and policies from a mental health facility, investigate criteria for use of physical restraints and monitoring protocols. Identify further data that are needed in order to draw accurate conclusions about this client.

2. Are this client's rights being violated?

Research the concept of client rights. Consider the physiologic as well as the psychologic impact of physical restraint on the client's rights. Review recommendations by the Joint Commission on Accreditation of Hospitals Organization (JCAHO) or other accrediting agencies related to use of restraints. Discuss when physical restraints are necessary to protect the safety of the client, other clients, or staff members.

3. What further data do you need in order to fairly evaluate the nurse's decision to place this client in restraints?

List further data that are needed on the basis of your research on accrediting recommendations or hospital policies. Consider data such as client assessment findings, comparison of this client's status with others who have required physical restraints, critical incident reports, and so on.

4. What are the advantages of delaying judgment or decisions about the use of physical restraints on this unit until all the facts are available?

Discuss the problems associated with drawing premature conclusions about any situation, even when the situation seems less than desirable. Consider how the use of physical restraints can be an emotional issue that may alter judgment. Identify the advantages of making decisions on the basis of accurate information.

5. What alternatives are there to placing clients in physical restraints?

Research other methods for dealing with combative clients, such as de-escalation, appropriate use of medications, and so on. Discuss how use of medications can also be considered a physical restraint. Identify countries that do not use physical restraints, such as England. Consider treatment methods used by those countries for client's who present a safety risk to themselves or others.

6. What risks do physical restraints pose to clients and staff members?

   Consider the physical and psychologic complications that may result from use of physical restraints, such as increased risk for skin injury, staff injury, and malpractice suits. Assess the need for staff training, the importance of documentation, and so on.

7. How can you apply the care of this client to other types of restrained clients?

   Recall instances in which you have encountered clients in physical restraints and the circumstances of each case. Identify possible complications for all clients who are restrained regardless of the reason for their confinement, such as skin alteration.

8. What attitude and cognitive critical thinking skills did you use for this case?

   Creativity, divergent thinking, clarification, faith in reason, and so on.

Mental Health Nursing
Schizophrenia

The client, a 45-year-old woman, was admitted to the crisis intervention unit at 10:00 AM after being picked up by the police. They found her wandering in and out of traffic on a busy city street. The crisis intervention unit has a maximum length of stay of 3 days. The client is a homeless person who is easily recognized by nursing staff members from previous admissions over the past 5 years. Her medical record from these admissions describe a 20-year history of schizophrenia. She has had multiple admissions for this problem and referrals for outpatient treatment. The client has taken a number of medications over the past 20 years, including chlorpromazine, perphenazine, and thiothixene. Her patient record does not identify any family. The unit assigned a case manager to her during her last admission 7 months ago. She has had no major medical illness but has been seen in the emergency department for minor illnesses and conditions, such as lacerations and respiratory infections.

The client is a thin woman who appears disheveled and dirty. She is wearing several layers of clothing even though it is summertime. Her hair is tangled. Her tongue protrudes repetitively, and she smacks her lips. She was cooperative during the admission interview and assessment, but at times she did not appear to understand the questions. Periodically she laughed for no apparent reason but did not say why she was laughing. She had no apparent injuries. She did complain of her feet hurting, and they appeared red, swollen, and dirty. Her shoes did not fit and had several holes. The client is 5 ft, 5 in tall and weighs 120 lbs. Her blood pressure is 135/80, her heart rate is 88 beats per minute (bpm), her respirations are 25 breaths per minute, and her oral temperature is 99.6F.

The client's diagnostic findings are as follows:

Hematology: RBC 4.6, Hgb 12 g/dL, Hct 37%, WBC 10,000

Urine Drug Screen: negative for illicit drugs

Urine culture and sensitivity: negative

Urinalysis: negative for glucose and ketones

~~~~

1. On the basis of the client's diagnostic data, what can you infer about the client's current mental status?

   Define any terms you do not understand. Separate relevant from irrelevant data. Cluster the data into related categories. Identify primary problems on the basis of the data clusters. Consider whether the problems you identified are based on the facts of the case, conjecture, or your feelings.

2. What further data are needed to confirm your inferences about the client's condition?

   From your data clusters, identify additional data that are needed to support the problems you identified. Consider information from the client's case manager; information about how and where she is obtaining medications; and her involvement with any community agencies, homeless shelters, and so on.

3. What are the client's priority problems and appropriate nursing diagnoses to address these problems?

   Consider the client's mental and physical status, including her hallucinations and delusions, hygiene, safety, and risk for infection. Identify the most appropriate nursing diagnosis by the North American Nursing Diagnosis Association (NANDA) for each of your identified problems. Prioritize these diagnoses according to the life-preservation framework or another prioritizing vehicle supplied by your school.

4. What nursing actions should you take to address the client's priority nursing diagnoses?

Research nursing actions for each of your identified priority nursing diagnoses. Consider the client's neurobiologic disorder of schizophrenia, as well as her physical problems. Decide which nursing activities would most effectively address the client's problems. Formulate short-term and long-term outcomes and determine how your nursing actions can help achieve those outcomes. Discuss the importance of discharge planning, identifying factors that failed in the past and whether the nurses believed their past interventions were effective.

5. What impact does the client's homelessness have on her current state?

Discuss the impact of deinstitutionalization on people such as the client, who may need the support afforded by long-term treatment centers. Consider the impact of homelessness on anyone, particularly those with mental disorders, including issues related to safety; exposure to human immunodeficiency virus (HIV); drug abuse; and physical problems due to poor nutrition, poor hygiene, inadequate medical treatment, and decreased ability to access psychiatric treatment.

6. How are chlorpromazine, perphenazine, and thiothixene used pharmacologically to treat schizophrenia?

Research each of the prescribed medications, noting their desired effects, mechanisms of action, and side effects. Identify the advantages and disadvantages of each, noting why one medication might be prescribed over another. Compare the side effects of these medications, identifying those that are associated with problems such as lip smacking or repetitive tongue protrusions. Explain how newly approved medications differ from older medications used for schizophrenia.

7. What is your opinion about the problem of homelessness in your community?

   Present your view of the homelessness problem in your community. Identify your biases, either negative or positive. Explain how your feelings could impact your care of people such as the client.

8. What attitude and cognitive critical thinking skills did you use to address this case?

   Divergent thinking, reasoning, clarification, intellectual humility, and so on.